1997

THE CHALLENGE OF ADOLESCENT HEALTH

Views from Catholic Social Teaching and the Social and Medical Sciences

Brenda W. Donnelly
Dennis M. Doyle
Una M. Cadegan
Teresa L. Thompson
Patricia Voydanoff
Joan McGuinness Wagner

University Press of America, Inc.
Lanham • New York • London

Copyright © 1997 by
University Press of America,® Inc.
4720 Boston Way
Lanham, Maryland 20706

3 Henrietta Street
London, WC2E 8LU England

Library of Congress Cataloging-in-Publication Data

The challenge of adolescent health : views from Catholic social
teaching and the social and medical sciences / Brenda Donnelly ... [et
al.]
p.   cm.
Includes bibliographical references and index.
1. Teenagers--Medical care--United States. 2. Teenagers--Medical
care--Religious aspects--Catholic church. 3. Teenagers--Health and
hygiene--United States. I. Donnelly, Brenda W.
RJ102.C46 1996   362.1'0835--dc20   96-35135 CIP

ISBN 0-7618-0560-5 (cloth: alk. ppr.)
ISBN 0-7618-0561-3 (pbk. : alk. ppr.)

CONTENTS

LIST OF TABLES AND FIGURES

PREFACE

Adolescence is a period of great risks, challenges, and opportunities. The second decade of life is characterized by physical, sexual, and psychological transformation from childhood to adulthood. For some, it brings with it unlimited enthusiasum, resiliency, and energy; for others it a period of confusion, trouble, and pain. Discusssion of policies and programs which impact the health and well-being of adolescents must integrate both the deheartening realities of the many risks to adolescent health and the restorative potential of the hope, knowledge, and commitment to the opportunities of the future.

This book provides a multi-disciplinary examination of the complex social issues surrounding adolescent health and health care delivery. It draws specifically on the resources of Catholic social teaching, presents an overview of the medical problems common among young people, and explores the social and familial contexts in which these problems arise. It provides a framework within which to view the conditions limiting the health and well-being of adolescents and to understand the resultant deterioration of the physical and mental health of adolescents in this country. The insights gained from Catholic social teaching are included with those of social science and medicine in order to formulate specific recommendations for creative and effective delivery of health care to adolescents.

INTENDED AUDIENCE

This book is intended as a resource for all professionals who work with adolescents and are concerned with their health and well-being. People of faith interested in proactive, morally consistent solutions to adolescent health issues will find this book very helpful. These constituencies include family physicians, pediatricians, school nurses, counselors, and those involved in youth or family ministries. Volunteers in community programs for young people, the administrators of Catholic hospitals, as well as

Catholic social service organizations and schools developing or utilizing programs for adolescents should find it helpful. This volume is intended for those who shape public policy and deliver health and human services to adolescents. It is also intended to broaden the understanding of those who focus their research efforts on adolescent development, the sociology of medicine, social or medical ethics, or Catholic social teaching. This book will have succeeded if it proves useful to any or all of the groups working to improve the health of adolescents.

OVERVIEW OF THE CONTENTS

This book deals specifically with the unique health needs of adolescents and focuses on the meaning of Catholic teaching as it is applied to those in the second decade of life. The writers explore the causes and consequences of common physical and mental health problems for adolescents. Because social conditions contribute in many cases at least as much to adolescent health problems as do the actual physical pathogens, this investigation extends well beyond the more traditional biomedical explorations. It deals with the unique health needs of adolescents and focuses on the meaning of Catholic teaching as it is applied to those in the second decade of life. Adolescent health needs are considered in light of Catholic teaching concerning the nature of the human person and of the ways in which people of faith are called to treat one another. We enumerate problems and limitations of health care delivery to adolescents and consider important policy issues that shape the current discourse concerning the health and well-being of young people. This book also provides specific suggestions for improving the health care of adolescents.

The first chapter summarizes the health concerns facing adolescents in the United States. An overview of the expected development of young people during adolescence is followed by an exploration of the meaning of health. The prevalence of various biomedical conditions, mental health problems, and social morbidities confronting adolescents is explored. The concomitants and clustering of these health conditions are discussed.

Chapter 2 considers the social context of adolescent health. Specific focus is applied to the role of the family in health and to the influence of mass media on adolescent health and health risking behaviors.

Chapter 3 addresses three important questions of adolescent health care from the teachings of the Catholic tradition. These questions --"Why health care?" "Why adolescent health care?" and "What type of health care?"-- provide a context within which our current system of health care services and any future systems can be evaluated.

The fourth chapter examines the delivery of health care to adolescents.

How the services are utilized as well as the identification of the barriers to effective use are considered in this section.

Chapter 5 explores some of the important issues in adolescent service delivery. The treatment and prevention of violence, early sexual activity, and the abuse of alcohol and other substances are examined. Parental involvement and adolescent autonomy are discussed and the most appropriate role of schools in health treatment and education is considered.

The final two chapters integrate relevant teachings from the Catholic faith with the understanding generated out of the social and medical perspectives to present suggestions for improving health care delivery to young people. Effective and morally consistent health care must focus on prevention of health problems. It must provide integrated care oriented to treating the whole person in the context of his/her family and community. Furthermore, it should encourage the use of age-appropriate health care services. In order to meet the challenge of adolescent health care in a manner consistent with the precepts of Christianity, such care must be family-centered, culturally-sensitive, and value-based.

Also provided are two additional tools for the reader. Chapter 7 summarizes the findings and implications of this work into general guidelines which can be used to develop, evaluate, and improve adolescent health care delivery. Lastly, the bibliography is extensive and broad. Those needing more detailed information about a specific condition, policy, argument, or program will find a wealth of information in these sources.

ACKNOWLEDGMENTS

The research for and writing of this document were made possible by generous funding from the Miller-Valentine-Walsh Fund. We are grateful to them for stimulating the project as well as for their continued support of the undertaking. We also appreciate the support provided by the University of Dayton. Brother Raymond L. Fitz, Father James Heft, and Dean Paul J. Morman were especially helpful in formulating the direction and focus of the project.

The integration of the insights gleaned from Catholic social teaching with those of demographers, physicians, and social scientists has been truly challenging. We have drawn on the learning of a diverse collection of individuals and organizations with a wide range of expertise, foci, and political agendas. A few of these sources hold some ideological positions inconsistent with those of Catholic social teaching, yet they provide important information and insight concerning the health and well-being of young people. Fortunately, we work in a community of scholars who understand the need for a multi-disciplinary approach to the complex social issues of the day. Adolescent health and health care delivery is one such complex and important issue.

Several years ago we began exploring the issues surrounding adolescent health and well-being through discussions with adolescent health care providers, ethicists, educators, and social service workers. These discussions were both stimulating and fruitful. We are grateful to all of those who participated in these discussions, especially Martha Carrick, Dr. Dean Berman, Dr. Jenny Davis-Berman, Dr. Patricia Dempsey, Doug McWan, Patty Martin, Linda Mercuri, Joan Place, Dr. Mary Pryor, Beth Roberts, Chris Sassonberg, Dr. Larry Ulrich, and Greg Way.

Helpful comments were received on an earlier draft of this document from Dr. Nancy Bell, Dr. James D. Robinson, and Dr. Patrick Sheeran. We also acknowledge the efforts of Vanessa Hsu, Lisa Thonnings, and Jennifer Westbrock who patiently located and collected information and resources for this work. Our work on this project was also aided greatly by the staff of the Roesch Library. We also want to thank Rebecca Ringenbach for her diligent editorial help in preparing this manuscript.

We have asked individuals to respond critically to early drafts of this document. Thorough, thoughtful, and beneficial reviews of an earlier draft were received from a number of scholars and practitioners with various areas of expertise. Among the reviewers, we found the comments of Dr. Susan M. Coupey, Dr. George D. Comerci, Dr. William Doherty, Dr. Melanie Gold, Mrs. Molly Kelly, Fr. Richard McCormick, Fr. Michael Place, Ms. Kathleen Sheeran, and Dr. and Mrs. John Willke to be especially helpful. In addition, some seventy individuals discussed and reviewed the book's guidelines and recommendations during a consultation held at the University of Dayton in May of 1995. While not all their suggestions found their way into this book, their input has resulted in a much improved document; we appreciate their efforts. Responsibility for the views presented in this book, however, rests solely with the authors.

Dayton, Ohio   Brenda W. Donnelly
August, 1996

INTRODUCTION

Almost no one would disagree that young people in the United States today are in a state of crisis. Fewer and fewer adolescents face the complexities of life with access to the support and services they need. The lives of more and more adolescents are in jeopardy because of the violence to which they are subjected, the risky behaviors in which they choose to engage, and the inaccessibility of appropriate medical care. Overburdened or otherwise ineffectual social institutions can no longer nurture, support, and protect young people as they did in the past. And as these institutions have become stretched, the physical and mental health of adolescents in this country has deteriorated.

As the medical community attempts to cope with the many and serious crises in adolescent health, health care professionals are exploring origins and causes in new and creative ways. Many have begun to realize that simple biomedical analysis insufficiently explains the causes of complex problems. As a consequence, an increasing number of health care professionals have been attempting to understand the problems of adolescent health as emerging from a social context. Social conditions contribute in some cases at least as much to adolescent health problems as do the actual physical pathogens; conversely, treating only the physical and medical may leave the underlying condition essentially untouched.

This development toward treating adolescents within their social and familial contexts should be applauded and encouraged. It raises a whole new set of challenges, however, because it requires an awareness of and a sensitivity to the values and standards that affect not only the physical health of individuals but also the institutional health of society. Addressing these new challenges requires drawing on all available resources. People of faith, in particular, will want to draw information and wisdom not only from the tools of science and medicine but also from what their own faith traditions tell them about the nature of the human person and the ways people are to treat one another.

To date, the Church, families, medical facilities, communities, and schools have devised largely reactive solutions to serious health and well-being issues facing adolescents. Perhaps instead these nurturing institutions might work at developing creative and proactive solutions to the health care needs of adolescents. To do this, their members will have to broach fundamental questions concerning the role that the Church, family and community should play in the lives of their youth. Developing these creative solutions will also require confronting the complexities of medical institutions and the relationships of these institutions with the individual adolescent, the family, and the community. Those working to take on this challenge must deal with questions, posit goals, and present models that provide needed medical care to adolescents within the context of their families and that strengthen adolescents' position in the community.

This project addresses these potentially daunting challenges by focusing on the health needs of adolescents, on their families, the medical establishment and the community. It draws specifically on the resources of the Christian tradition, including the insights of the Gospels and of Roman Catholic social teaching, for a framework within which to view both the seriousness of the problems and the possibility of solutions. Finally, it attempts to formulate some specific recommendations for creative and effective delivery of health care to adolescents.

CHAPTER 1

HEALTH PROBLEMS OF AMERICAN ADOLESCENTS

This report presumes, as many people working in the area already know, that adolescent health is affected by a variety of interconnected factors. Accordingly, we begin with definitions of adolescence and of health that attempt to be both specific and inclusive; that is, to capture the complexity of the situation without being overly general. This broad definition of health then leads to a discussion of adolescent health problems that includes not only those contracted inadvertently but also those more or less consciously chosen, not only diseases but also destructive behaviors, with origins not only biomedical but also social. A discussion of how a variety of sociodemographic factors affect these problems and conditions, and the interrelationships among them, concludes the first section of this report.

ADOLESCENCE DEFINED

Adolescence refers to the social, physical, and psychological transition from childhood to adulthood. Generally this transition occurs after age 10; research on adolescence usually focuses on 10- to 19-year olds. During this period, growth and development are dramatic. Approximately 20% of adult height and 50% of adult weight are gained during adolescence (Strasburger, 1989). The second decade of life is a time not only of drastic physical but also behavioral change. Most fundamental of these changes is the onset of puberty--a biological change--but many cognitive, emotional, psychological and social changes occur during these years as well (Elkind, 1992; Johnson, 1989).

These changes and developments occur over the course of the teen years at many different rates and are influenced by a host of cultural, economic, and historical conditions (Kreipe & Sahler, 1991). While puberty generally occurs near the beginning of adolescence, adult brain development and the social maturity that accompanies it generally do not follow for another five or six years (Hamburg, 1992).

Because adolescents are often more mature physically than mentally or emotionally, they are often ill-prepared to make the serious decisions they face. As they explore the world and try to discover their place in it, they are often unaware of the risks their behaviors involve. As David Hamburg points out, adolescents:

> resemble a larger version of toddlers--having the newly acquired capacity to get into all sorts of novel and risky situations, but all too little judgement and information on which to base decisions about how to handle themselves. (Hamburg, 1992: 183)

Adolescence is generally divided into three stages: early, middle, and late. The exact age ranges are arbitrary and approximate. They are meant to identify common tendencies among young people as they develop from children to adults. With some consistency, adolescents experience changes in their physical, psychological, social, and moral circumstances (Felice, 1992). The delivery of adequate health care to adolescents presupposes an understanding of these patterns of growth and the developmental tasks associated with each phase. They are summarized in Table 1.1.

In the first stage of adolescence, ages 10 to 13 years, young people experience the most rapid phase of pubertal development. They develop primary and secondary sex characteristics and often grow two to five inches each year (Felice, 1992; Gander & Gardiner, 1981). Sometimes the growth of hands and feet outpaces the growth of the rest of the body causing clumsiness and awkwardness. During this stage adolescents must adjust to a very new body which often causes increasing self-consciousness (Sahler & McAnarney, 1981; Stevens-Simon & Reichert, 1994). Often adolescents in the early stage of development become obsessed with their own behavior and appearance and begin to assume (often incorrectly) that they are the focus of other people's attention as well[1] (Elkind, 1992; Gander & Gardiner,1981). Furthermore, because they see themselves as the focus of everyone's attention, they often conclude that they are unique, invulnerable,

---

[1]   This results in what David Elkind refers as to young teenagers' tendency to "construct an 'imaginary audience,' a belief that everyone in their immediate vicinity is watching them, thinking about them, and interested in their every thought and action. This imaginary audience gives rise to a heightened sense of self-consciousness unique to early adolescence when the audience is most powerful" (Elkind, 1992: 26).

TABLE 1.1: Growth Tasks of Adolescence by Developmental Phase

Tasks:	Independence	Body Image	Career Plans	Sexual Drives	Relationships	Value System	Conceptualization
Early Adolescence: 10 to 13 Years	Breaks emotionally from parents and prefers friends to family	Adjustment to pubescent changes; Increasing self-conciousness	Vague and even unrealistic plans	Sexual curiosity	Unisexual peer group; adult crushes	Drop in superego; Testing of moral systems of parents	Concrete Thinking Development of the "imaginary audience" and a "personal fable"
Middle Adolescence:	Ambivalence about separation	"Trying on" different images to find real self		Sexual experimentation;opposite sex viewed as sex object	Beginning of heterosexual peer group; Multiple adult role models	Self-centered	Fascinated by new capacity for thinking
Late Adolescence: 17 Years and Older	Integration of independence issues	Integration of a satisfying body image with personality	Specific goals and steps to implement them	Beginning of intimacy and caring	Individual reltaionships more important than peer group	Idealism; rigid concepts of right and wrong. Altruism; asceticism.	Ability to abstract; Decresing importance of the"imaginary audience" and "personal fable"

SOURCE: Adapted from Felice, 1992, Adolescence, pp. 65-73 in *Developmental-behavioral pediatrics*, edited by Levine, Carey, & Crocker: 69 (Table 6-2), copyright W. B. Saunders Co.; and Elkind, 1992, Cognitive development, pp. 24-26 in *Comprehensive adolescent health care*, edited by Friedman, Fisher, & Schonberg, copyright Appleton & Lange.

invincible, and for all intents and purposes, immortal (Elkind, 1992). It is this "personal fable", the belief that they are invulnerable to harm, that encourages many early-stage-adolescents to engage in health-compromising and risky behaviors (Elkind, 1992).

Middle adolescence includes those who are aged approximately 14 through 16. Physical growth and weight gain continue through this stage. Average weight gain between the ages of 11 and 16 is 42 pounds for girls and 56 pounds for boys (Gander & Gardiner, 1981). Characteristically, those who are in this stage of adolescence are beginning to realize that they are not entirely unique and that not everyone is interested in watching them (Gander & Gardiner, 1981). Young people in this stage of development begin to develop their capacity for abstract reasoning. They become capable of introspection and often stretch their mental abilities by pondering hypothetical situations. Some become fascinated with their new found ability to consider multiple solutions to different problems.

During this stage adolescents also work to establish their own identity by loosening their emotional ties to their parents and siblings (Sahler & McAnarney, 1981; Stevens-Simon & Reichert, 1994). This period is often characterized by a shift from intense friendships with those of the same sex to more male-female interactions (Gander & Gardiner, 1981). "The cognitive changes of puberty make many middle adolescents defiant, narcissistic, and self-reliant" (Stevens-Simon & Reichert, 1994: 24).

The third stage of adolescence begins at about age 17. By the time they reach late adolescence, most young people have adjusted to their changed bodies and increased cognitive capabilities (Sahler & McAnarney, 1981). They are able to consider problems systematically and abstractly; what Piaget refers to as "formal operations" are developed for many during this stage. Those without formal operations are only able to discuss the world as it is while those who have developed to this stage of cognitive development are able to discuss the world *as it might become* (Clarke-Stewart & Koch, 1983:379). As Felice points out:

(t)he social implications of this stage of cognitive development are many. Older adolescents can be avid conversationalists with opinions on every issue. In addition, adolescents can now see a host of alternatives to parents' and may promptly point these out to a beleaguered mother or father. (Felice, 1992: 68)

Adolescents in the third stage of development are capable of considering the future with some degree of realism. Much of their energy is devoted to establishing their place in the adult world both in terms of their career and in establishing more long-term personal relationships. The value system within which this planning takes place is characteristically somewhat more rigid than that of adults and accompanied by idealism and an increasing sense of altruism. In addition, youth in this stage of development :

> can generally shed the strong need for a peer group in favor of a close, intimate, and caring relationship. For many young persons, finding a partner or significant other becomes a major search; this is the typical age for falling in love. (Felice, 1992: 69)

Successful progression through each of the developmental tasks of adolescence is necessary for healthy adulthood.

DEFINITION OF HEALTH

Most large-scale evaluations of the health of adolescents in the United States are based on a broad definition of adolescent health. For example, the U.S. Congress' Office of Technology Assessment (1991a) uses a multifaceted definition. Health is seen not only as the presence or absence of physical disease and disability, but also as the absence of health-compromising behaviors such as drug use, smoking, and early sexual activity. Health is also measured in terms of social competence--whether or not the adolescent is dealing well with the day-to-day difficulties of reaching adulthood. The current project uses this broad approach to delineate adolescent health issues. In this document, then, health is more than simply the absence of disease. Following the World Health Organization's definition, "health is a state of complete physical, mental and social well-being and not merely the absence of disease or infirmity" (Polgar, 1968: 330).

There are a number of ways to establish health or illness among different groups in a society. Morbidity and mortality statistics offer rough estimates of the health of adolescents. Measures such as physicians' diagnoses, hospitalization rates, death rates, police reports, and statistics from schools and social service agencies are all useful and necessary indicators of various aspects of adolescent health (Gans, Blyth, Elster, & Gaveras, 1990; Gans, McManus, & Newacheck, 1991).

There are, however, difficulties involved in the interpretation of each of these measures for the adolescent population. For example, the age categories are often not consistent from one study to another. Whenever possible, data in this report focus on 10- to 19-year olds but sometimes the information is available for only a portion of this group or includes young people in their early twenties. Furthermore, the comprehensiveness of mortality and morbidity statistics varies from state to state. For example, in 1990 only 32 states required health care professionals to report cases of

HIV infection (United States Congress, Office of Technology Assessment, 1991b). Even more problematic are the available measures of health-compromising behaviors such as substance abuse, early sexual activity, and violence. Crime and victimization statistics vary greatly from jurisdiction to jurisdiction; some argue that they may more reliably reflect the recording procedures of the police department than actual delinquent behavior. Often the data do not include variations by income, race, or other social conditions, thereby limiting our ability to identify the underlying conditions which place some adolescents at higher risk for ill-health than others. Taken in concert, however, the available data allow an understanding of adolescent health problems and allow one to gauge the overall well-being of teenagers in the United States.

TYPES OF HEALTH PROBLEMS

Because adolescence is a period of rapid physical and psychosocial growth and development, the health problems experienced by adolescents are somewhat different from those of other age groups. While on the whole adolescents experience relatively low rates of cancer, hypertension, and other physical disorders, they are subject to a number of unique developmental conditions and they are more likely than other groups to engage in a number of risk-taking behaviors that seriously threaten their health (Runyan & Gerken, 1991; Gans, McManus, & Newacheck, 1991). Unlike those in other age groups, the principal causes of adolescent death and illness are largely preventable. Accidents, homicide, suicide, substance abuse, and the consequences of early sexual activity are the major causes of mortality and morbidity among adolescents (Hamburg, 1992: 230). Figure 1. 1 shows that nearly 75% of adolescent deaths can be accounted for by three largely preventable causes of death: accidents, suicide, and homicide (Fingerhut & Kleinman, 1989; Millstein & Litt, 1990; National Center for Health Statistics, 1984). Because of the relative prevalence of death by these three causes, adolescents and young adults were the only age groups in the United States whose death rates *rose* between 1960 and 1980 (Hamburg, 1989; Fingerhut & Kleinman, 1989).

　　This report divides adolescent health problems into three major types: biomedical or physiologic conditions, mental health problems, and social morbidity among adolescents. Research reveals that the largely preventable social morbidities are by far the greatest threat to adolescent health and well-being. Thus, any approach to adolescent health care not only must take into account the biomedical and mental health problems distinctive to adolescence, but also must give special attention to those medical problems resulting from social conditions and risk-taking behaviors.

FIGURE 1.1:   Death Rates Among Adolescents by Accidents, Suicide, Homicide and Diseases by Age in Years

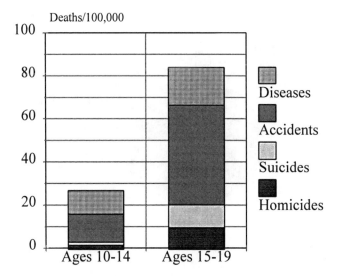

SOURCE: Fingerhut & Kleinman, 1989. Trends in current status in childhood mortality United States, 1900-85. *Vital & Health Statistics Series 3*: 20.

Biomedical Health Problems: Nondevelopmental

Like people in all age groups, teenagers are subject to a variety of acute and chronic conditions that adversely affect their health (Gans, McManus, & Newacheck, 1991). As can be seen in Figure 1.2, most often adolescents visit physicians for a variety of relatively minor acute conditions. These conditions (colds and sore throats, ear infections, hay fever and allergy, skin problems, and vision disorders, etc.) account for nearly a quarter of all visits to the physician by adolescents (Nelson, 1991; Gans, McManus, & Newacheck, 1991).

     Fairly clear estimates of the number of adolescents who suffer from chronic physical ailments have been derived from a representative national

FIGURE 1.2:   Most Common Diagnoses for Adolescents' Visits to
                    Physicians, 1985.

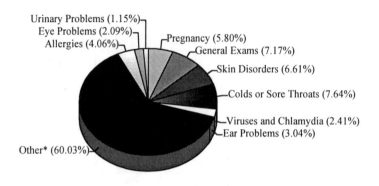

* Each totalling less than 1% of the diagnoses

SOURCE: Adapted from Nelson, 1991, Advance Data from Vital and Health
            Statistics of the National Center for Health Statistics, U.S.
            Department of Health and Human Services, Number 196, April 11,
            1991: 5.

survey concerning 7,465 adolescents 10 to 17 years old[2] (Newacheck,
McManus & Fox, 1991). Nearly one third--31.5%--of the adolescent
population under 18 suffer from at least one condition which lasts at least
three months. According to these data, approximately 8.6 million 10- to 17-
year-olds have at least one chronic physical condition, nearly 2 million have
two, and 875,000 are estimated to have three or more chronic physical

---

[2]   These data were derived from the 1988 National Health Interview Survey,
        Child Health Supplement.

conditions (Newacheck, McManus & Fox, 1991; Westbrook & Stein, 1994). Other data suggest that approximately two million or 5-10% of adolescents experience a chronic physiologic condition, such as leukemia,cerebral palsy, diseases of the musculoskeletal system, or a hearing impairment, that *markedly* limits their activities (Gans, Blyth, Elster, & Gaveras, 1990; Newacheck, 1989a; United States Congress Office of Technology Assessment, 1991b; Millstein & Litt, 1990). Diseases of the respiratory system account for more than one-fifth of the chronic illnesses among adolescents (Millstein & Litt, 1990). Approximately 13% of all adolescents suffer from respiratory allergies (Westbrook & Stein, 1994). Table 1.2 displays current estimates of chronic conditions in American adolescents.

Biomedical Health Problems: Developmental

Some chronic health problems are tied directly to the hormonal changes and rapid growth which are characteristic of the second decade of life. These occur more frequently among adolescents than other age groups. Scoliosis, Osgood-Schlatter disease, and slipped capital femoral epiphysis (skeletal disorders), are associated with the rapid growth of adolescence (Millstein & Litt, 1990). Similarly, dysmenorrhea (painful menstrual cycles) is a frequently reported difficulty for young women and the leading medical cause of school absenteeism among female teens (Brookman, 1989a; DuRant, 1991; Gans, Blyth, Elster & Gaveras, 1990; Litt, 1987; Millstein & Litt, 1990). Because of the effects of menstrual blood loss and inadequate dietary intake, females in middle adolescence are more likely than other women to suffer from problems associated with iron deficiency (Vaughan & Litt, 1990b). Some vision problems are also attributed to the rapid growth of facial bones and orbits during puberty (Greydanus & Hofmann, 1989a; Vaughan & Litt, 1990b).

Acne, a disorder of the sebaceous glands, is another developmental condition which constitutes a health problem for many adolescents. In fact, most American adolescents experience acne. Approximately 90% of adolescent males and 80% of adolescent females are affected with acne to some degree (Greydanus & Hofmann, 1989b). For many adolescents, this condition is more than an annoyance: many are left with disfiguring scars. While acne is not life-threatening, approximately $120 million is spent annually to treat it (Wagner & Wagner, 1985; Greydanus & Hofmann, 1989b).

TABLE 1.2:   Prevalence Estimates of Chronic Physiologic
Conditions in Adolescents

General Condition Category	Cases/1000 U.S. Adolescents
Musculoskeletal impairments	20.9
Deafness and hearing loss	17.0
Blindness and visual impairments	16.0
Speech defects	18.9
Cerebral Palsy	1.2[*]
Diabetes	1.5[*]
Sickle cell disease	0.9[*]
Anemia	5.8
Asthma	46.8
Respiratory allergies	130.3
Eczema and skin allergies	35.2
Epilepsy and seizures	3.3
Arthritis	8.7
Heart Disease	17.4
Frequent or repeated ear infections	33.6
Frequent diarrhea/bowel trouble	9.6
Digestive allergies	21.1
Frequent or severe headaches	45.8
Other	30.0

[*] Relative Standard Error exceeds 30% of estimate value.

SOURCE: Newacheck, McManus & Fox, Prevalence and Impact of Chronic
Illness Among Adolescents, *American Journal of Diseases of
Children*, vol. 145, 1991: 1370, Table 4. Copyright 1991, American
Medical Association.

Young people with developmental conditions are often encountered by pediatricians treating adolescents:

John was fairly typical. He was 15 years old and wanted to begin working. Required to have a physical, he came for his first one in five years. It revealed that he had moderately severe scoliosis and severe acne. He was referred to an orthopedist for treatment of his back and was given a prescription for his acne.

... and Cara, a 14 year old, was referred by a school nurse after fainting in school. Her history was that her menses had begun during the past year and she had experienced constant vaginal bleeding for the prior three months. She had been secretive about the bleeding and assumed that it was normal. A complete hematological workup revealed no pathologic cause but a severe iron deficiency from the chronic blood loss.

    Treatment included iron replacement, progesterone medication to counteract the unopposed estrogen bleeding, and an explanation and education for the patient and her mother. It was explained that ovulation often does not occur regularly during early sexual maturation and that without ovulation, the hormone progesterone is not produced. The estrogen hormone constantly stimulates the endometrium which then bleeds unchecked.

Sam's asthma brought him to the teen clinic office fairly frequently throughout his teen years. On one of his visits he confided that he was worried that he was different from "everybody else." He thought that perhaps his growth and development were slower than they should be and that he had a lot of leg pain after exercise. He admitted that he sometimes avoided the prescribed asthma regime because he didn't want his friends to know he was "a sicky" and because he thought that it probably caused his acne.

    I tried to carefully address his concerns and reassure him that his development was normal for his age and that the leg pains he suffered were also nothing out of the ordinary for a growing youth. Once he learned that his skin problems were unrelated to his medication, he began to take his medication more consistently.

SOURCE: Mary Pryor, M.D., letter to the authors, August, 1995.

Mental Health Problems

Nearly one third of the two million adolescents suffering from debilitating chronic illnesses suffer from some sort of psychological disorder (Millstein & Litt, 1990). Diagnosable mental disorders including attention deficit disorders, conduct disorders, anxiety, and depression affect between 18 and 22% of adolescents (United States Congress logy Assessment, 1991a, 1991b). Much higher percentages of adolescents report subjective distress; for example, in the 1987 National Adolescent Student Health Survey, 61% of 8th and 10th graders reported feeling sad and hopeless sometimes or often during the previous month (American School Health Association, et al., 1989; Gans, Blyth, Elster, & Gaveras, 1990; United States Congress logy Assessment, 1991b).

One of the more serious and prevalent psychological disorders among adolescents is depression. The symptoms of depression among adolescents are similar to those among adults. These individuals report feeling helpless, say that they have nothing to look forward to, suffer from fatigue or insomnia, and lose the ability to concentrate for long periods (Saxe, Cross & Silverman, 1986). Some argue that the high rate of depression among teens is tied to the social pressures they encounter as they try to make decisions concerning their careers, marriage, and childbearing and to assume the other responsibilities of adulthood (Vaughan & Litt, 1990d). In one national study, more than a third of the young women and 15% of the adolescent men reported often feeling "sad and hopeless" while even higher proportions said that it was hard for them to deal with all the stress and difficult situations in their lives (American School Health Association, et al., 1989; Dryfoos, 1990b).

Social Morbidities

Many adolescents experience physical and mental problems that are not strictly biomedical in origin. These "social morbidities"[3] are rooted directly in the social environment of the adolescent: the conditions under which they live and the behaviors in which they have chosen to participate[4]

---

[3]   Some researchers refer to this complex of health problems as the "new morbidity." See for example, Haggerty, Roghmann, and Pless (1993) and Baumeister, Kupstas, and Klindworth (1991).

[4]   Because most estimates of social morbidities rely on school-based assessments, their prevalence is often underestimated; health-compromising

(Baumeister, Kupstas, & Klindworth, 1991; Gans, McManus, & Newacheck, 1991; Haggerty, Roghmann, & Pless, 1993; Lavin, Shapiro, & Weill, 1992).

Adolescents frequently participate in behaviors that place their health at risk or impair their social competence. Often called risk-taking or health-compromising behaviors, they often involve some decision to participate on the part of the teen. Risk-taking behaviors relatively common among adolescents include early sexual activity; use of alcohol, tobacco, and drugs; violence; and school failure and dropping out (Gans, Blyth, Elster, & Gaveras, 1990; Blum, 1987a; Donovan & Jessor, 1985; Dryfoos, 1990b; Werner, 1991). Indeed, most adolescent deaths are tied directly to risk-taking behaviors: accidental injuries, suicide, and homicide (Fingerhut & Kleinman, 1989; Ginsberg & Loffredo, 1993; Blum, 1987a; Runyan & Gerken, 1989, 1991; United States Congress logy Assessment, 1991a).

Social morbidities also include health problems which go beyond the decisions adolescents make and are tied more directly with their social environments. Teens who attend schools or live in neighborhoods where violence is common may be *subjected* to assault or intimidation without ever having *decided* to participate in health-compromising behaviors (Ginsberg & Loffredo, 1993). Early sexual activity is often coercive on the part of at least one partner; young people who are subject to rape, incest, or other forms of coercive sexual activity do not *decide* to participate in this risky behavior. Similarly, adolescents who drive substandard cars without air bags, functional seat belts, or decent tires may be *subjected* to an increased likelihood of injury by the sheer consequence of their limited resources even if they make every effort to drive safely. Television, movies, and the printed media provide a cultural context which is, at best, generally not health-promoting. It may serve to promote health-compromising behaviors such as alcohol consumption, smoking, and nonmarital sexual activity. Similarly, poverty and racism directly impact the ability of some youth to lead healthy, socially competent lives; the health problems associated with these conditions are not strictly biomedical yet neither are they the result of the adolescents' decisions to participate in risky behaviors.

---

behaviors of those not in school are even more common than among youth enrolled in schools. See Grunbaum & Basen-Engquist (1993), for a comparison of health-compromising behaviors of students enrolled in a regular high school with those of students enrolled at a dropout prevention/dropout recovery high school.

Accidental Injuries

As can be seen in Figure 1.1 (page 9), accidental injuries to adolescents are responsible for more than half of all teen deaths (United States Congress logy Assessment, 1991b: 117).   Figure 1.3 presents a breakdown of these accidental deaths.   More than three quarters stem from accidents involving vehicles (cars, trucks, all-terrain vehicles, bicycles and motorcycles). Drowning accounts for about 8% of accidental deaths.   Since the United States has the most heavily armed civilian population in history, it is not surprising that another 3.9% of the accidental deaths among teens

FIGURE 1.3:   Accidental Injury Deaths By Cause Among U.S. Adolescents, Ages 10 to 19, 1992.

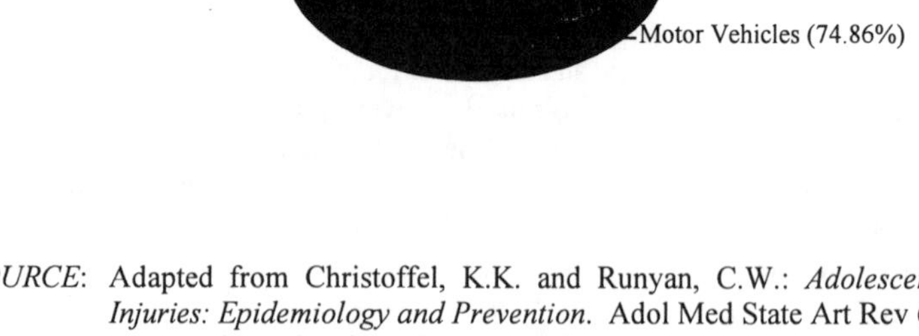

SOURCE: Adapted from Christoffel, K.K. and Runyan, C.W.: *Adolescent Injuries: Epidemiology and Prevention.*   Adol Med State Art Rev 6: Foreword, Hanley & Belfus, Philadelphia, 1995, with permission.

are due to the misuse of firearms[5] (Adelson, 1992; Cohall & Cohall, 1995; Sloan, Kellerman, Reay, Ferris, Koepsell, Rivara, Rice, Gray, & LoGerfo, 1988; United States Congress, Office of Technology Assessment, 1991b).

Information on nonfatal injuries to adolescents is difficult to find. It can be safely assumed, however, that for every fatal injury a large number of nonfatal accidents also occur; one study estimates that there are more than 1000 injuries for every motor vehicle death among people aged 10 to 20 (Li, Baker & Frattaroli, 1995). Motor vehicle and recreational vehicle accidents, for instance, are the most frequently cited cause of hospitalization for 12- to 17-year olds (Millstein & Litt, 1990).

Sports and recreational activities are also a leading cause of nonfatal accidental injury (United States Congress Office of Technology Assessment, 1991b; Paulson, 1990). In 1988 the Consumer Product Safety Commission reported that when one focuses on accidents involving purchased equipment and excludes motor vehicle and firearm accidents, injuries resulting from sports activities account for the four most common causes of emergency room visits for 10- to 18-year olds. Nineteen percent of those visits can be attributed to playing basketball. Football injuries account for 18.6% of these visits, followed by bicycle accidents (14.3%), and baseball accidents (8.7% [United States Congress Office of Technology Assessment, 1991b: 122]). Among athletic activities, however, football is probably one of the most hazardous (United States Congress Office of Technology Assessment, 1991b, Paulson, 1990). In one recent study of high school athletes, 61% of the football players were injured at least moderately during the course of the year (McLain & Reynolds, 1989). In an earlier study 80% of high school football players were injured and fewer than one death per 100,000 participants was expected during the course of the year (Kraus & Conroy, 1984).

Substance Abuse

Figure 1.4 presents the results of a national survey on substance abuse among adolescents. It illustrates that a great number of adolescents have used illicit substances at some time during their lives. The substances used by these young people include the whole range of illicit drugs from heroin and cocaine to tobacco and alcohol. Some of the most frequently used

---

[5] The deaths by homicide and suicide involving the use of a handgun are not included in this figure. Overall, gunshot wounds are the third leading cause of unintentional injury deaths among those aged 10 to 19. Between 1982 and 1988, nearly 3000 adolescents died from firearm injuries (*Morbidity and Mortality Weekly Report*, 1992).

FIGURE 1.4:   Percent of 12- to 17-Year-Olds Using Different Types of Substances During Lifetime, 1988

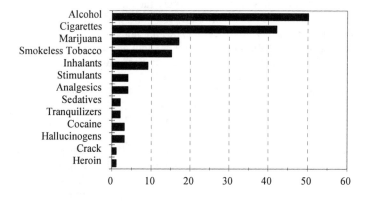

SOURCE: National Institute on Drug Abuse, *Highlights of the 1988 National Survey on Drug Abuse*: 62.

substances are discussed here.

According to the National Institute on Drug Abuse, over half of the 12- to 17-year olds have consumed alcohol (National Institute on Drug Abuse, 1990) while among high school seniors alcohol consumption appears much higher[6] (92% [Johnston, O'Malley, & Bachman, 1988]). This drinking is typically not done in "moderation" (Rogers & Adger, 1993). According to researchers of the National Institute for Drug Abuse, 30% of high school seniors, 23% of tenth graders, and 13% of eighth graders report drinking five or more drinks at least twice a month (Johnston, O'Malley, & Bachman, 1991). Some of these adolescents are alcoholics[7] and reflect all of the

---

[6]   These data do not include teenagers who are no longer attending school. It is reasonable to expect that those who have dropped out of high school are even more likely than high school seniors to regularly consume alcohol, smoke tobacco or marijuana, or use cocaine (*Morbidity and Mortality Weekly Report*, March 4, 1994).

[7]   According to the National Council on Alcoholism and Drug Dependencies (NCADD) and the American Society of Addiction Medicine (ASAM),

behavioral and physiological problems associated with the disease. Adolescents who drink alcohol and are pregnant also subject their babies to a wide spectrum of alcohol-related difficulties including fetal alcohol syndrome (Rogers & Adger, 1993).

While some adolescents do suffer directly from alcohol use, some of the most pressing problems associated with alcohol consumption result from its lessening the analytic capabilities of the drinker. Because of alcohol's tendency to decrease the user's inhibitions and to slow the user's reactions, its use is an important factor for all types of accidents. About one fifth of all adolescent deaths are from alcohol-related car accidents (National Commission Against Drunk Driving, 1988). This means that about half of the motor vehicle crash fatalities among adolescents ages 15 to 19 are related to alcohol (National Commission Against Drunk Driving, 1988). Alcohol is involved in close to 40% of adolescent drownings and 40% of homicide victims between the ages of 15 and 24 had been drinking alcohol shortly before their death (Runyan & Gerken, 1991). Early sexual activity is also related to alcohol use (Foster, 1986).

As both Figures 1.4 and 1.5 show, tobacco is another commonly used drug. Researchers estimate that 11% of high school seniors smoked at least a half-pack of cigarettes each day (O'Malley, Johnston, & Bachman, 1993). Although it is illegal in the United States to sell cigarettes to minors, 8.5 million adolescents 17 and under (42%) report smoking cigarettes and over 3 million (15%) have used smokeless tobacco (National Institute on Drug Abuse, 1990; National Institute on Drug Abuse, 1989a). Smoking among adolescents is, in fact, a common health risk for teenagers in many nations (Amos, 1991; Roosmalen & McDaniel, 1992; Stanton & Silva, 1991). A recent national survey of adolescents reports that 72% of adolescents have experimented with cigarette smoking (Escobedo, Marcus, Holtzman, & Giovino, 1993). Researchers have found that even infrequent experimentation with cigarettes greatly increases the likelihood of becoming a smoker in adulthood and that the use of tobacco is associated with increased rates of cancer, emphysema, bronchitis, and heart disease (Chassin, Presson, Sherman, & Edwards, 1990; Moss, Allen, Giovino, & Mills, 1992; Slade, 1993). It is important for adolescents to realize,

---

"Alcoholism is a primary, chronic disease with genetic, psychosocial, and environmental factors influencing its development and manifestations. The disease is often progressive and fatal. It is characterized by continuous or periodic impaired control over drinking; preoccupation with the drug, alcohol; use of alcohol despite adverse consequences; and distortions in thinking, most notably denial." (Morse & Flavin, 1992: 1013; see also, Flavin & Morse, 1991; Rogers & Adger, 1993).

FIGURE 1.5:   Percent of 12- To 17-Year-Olds' Substance Use in
Lifetime, In Past Year, and in Past Month, 1988

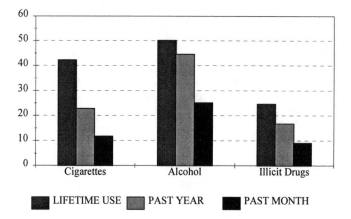

SOURCE: National Institute on Drug Abuse, *Highlights of the 1988 National
Household Survey on Drug Abuse*: 62-63.

however, that while:

> . . . most complications of tobacco use are reserved for adulthood, a
> striking array of problems can develop soon after regular tobacco use
> becomes established.   Cough, sputum production, and dyspnea on
> exertion are common symptoms among young people who smoke. Gum
> recession, leukoplakia, and even malignant oral lesions are frequent in
> moist-snuff users. (Slade, 1993: 307)

This author goes on to point out that tobacco smoke is responsible for a
large proportion of low birth weight infants born to adolescent mothers and
that cigarettes are a primary cause of deadly fires in this country (Slade,
1993; McGuire, 1989).

Adolescents' illicit drug use also extends to marijuana, cocaine,
anabolic/androgenic steroids, tranquilizers, a full range of inhalants, and
hallucinogens such as LSD or PCP.   Estimates derived from a 1991
nationally representative sample indicate that 44% of all high school seniors
reported using an illicit substance before graduation (O'Malley, Johnston,
& Bachman, 1993). According to one national survey, marijuana is the
most commonly abused of these drugs: approximately 3.5 million (17%)
12- to 17-year olds have tried marijuana (National Institute on Drug Abuse,

1990; National Institute on Drug Abuse, 1989b). Some 2.9% of the nation's 12- to 17-year olds have used cocaine and almost as many (2.8%) have used a hallucinogen in the past year (National Institute on Drug Abuse, 1990).

The use of illicit substances places these adolescents at higher risk of addiction, physical problems, delinquency, depression, involvement in crime and HIV infection (Baumrind, 1987; Gans, Blyth, Elster, & Gaveras, 1990). Habitual substance abuse during adolescence leads to arrested cognitive and moral development which sometimes extends long beyond recovery into adulthood (Nowinski, 1990).

Early Sexual Activity
Another important social behavior with adverse health consequences is the early sexual activity of teenagers. Adolescents are becoming sexually active (i.e. they have experienced coitus at least once), at increasingly earlier ages. As Figure 1.6 illustrates, by the time they reach their senior year in high school, a majority of the nearly 12,000 students surveyed by the Centers for Disease Control report having had sexual intercourse (Centers for Disease Control, 1992). Over recent years, population surveys document similar rates of sexual activity among young women in the United States. Figures from the Centers for Disease Control, for example, indicate that in 1988, 25.6% of 15 year-olds, more than half (51%) of surveyed 17 year-olds, and three quarters of 19 year-olds (75.3%) reported having had premarital sexual intercourse[8] (*Morbidity and Mortality Weekly Report*, 1991b; National Longitudinal Survey of Youth, 1983).

According to these data and those from the National Longitudinal Survey of Youth, young men tend to initiate sexual activity somewhat earlier than do young women but by late adolescence the percentage of sexually active girls more closely approximates that of boys[9](Centers for

---

[8] These data are based on the adolescent respondents from a survey of 8450 women 15-44 years conducted by the Centers for Disease Control's National Center for Health Statistics.

[9] There is evidence to suggest, however, that adolescent males probably exaggerate their sexual experiences in self-report surveys. If, as estimated by self-report data, some 5 million teenaged males are sexually active--and the births and abortions arising from liasons between adlut males and adolescent girls are considered--then the number pf births and abortions attributed to the female partners of these young men would far exceed those currently seen (Males, 1993).

FIGURE 1. 6:   Percent of Sexually Active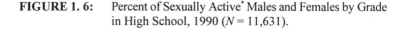 Males and Females by Grade in High School, 1990 (*N* = 11,631).

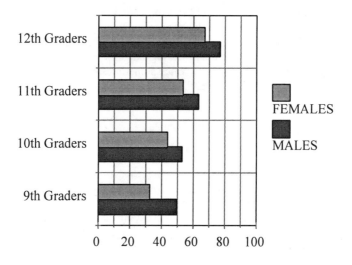

*Ever experienced sexual intercourse preceding the survey.

SOURCE: Centers for Disease Control, Youth Risk Behavior Survey, 1990, *Morbidity and Mortality Weekly Report*, 1992: Table 1, page 886.

Disease Control, 1992; Hayes, 1987).

Adolescents who engage in sexual activity at a young age place themselves at high risk for becoming infected with a sexually transmitted disease. There is evidence that adolescent women, because of the unique physiological conditions of their age, are more likely to be infected by various STD's if exposed to pathogens (Kipke & Hein, 1990). While their sexual activity is often sporadic, teens tend to change sexual partners more frequently than older couples, thus placing themselves at higher risk of sexually transmitted diseases (Boyer, 1990). Teenagers, in part because of their sense of invulnerability and in part because they lack sufficient understanding of physiology and pathology, tend to believe that they will never become infected. Furthermore, adolescents:

> . . .apparently to a greater extent than adults tend to have spontaneous rather than premeditated sex. Without a prior acknowledgement that

coitus may occur, preventative actions are hindered. Moreover, teenagers, like older persons, are awkward when communicating about sexuality, whether with the opposite sex or with their health care provider. This combination of denying the possibility of exposure and avoiding discussion of the consequences increases the likelihood that sexually active teenagers will acquire and/or transmit STDs. (Cates, 1990: 419)

Their chances of contracting a STD are also higher than that of adults because adolescents are relatively "poor" users of barrier methods of artificial contraception, which provide at least some protection against infection[10] (Sikand & Fisher, 1992).

Sexually transmitted diseases are at epidemic levels among adolescents; some 3 million adolescents contract a STD each year (Braverman, 1996; *Facts at a Glance*, January 1992; Gans, Blyth, Elster, & Gaveras, 1990; Kulig, 1996). If left untreated, many of these diseases are very serious and have consequences such as infertility, ectopic pregnancy, pelvic inflammatory disease, urethritis, meningitis, carcinoma, dysentery, and arthritis (Schydlower & Shafer, 1990; United States Congress Office of Technology Assessment, 1991b). There is also reason to believe that individuals with sexually transmitted diseases such as syphilis or herpes may be more likely to contract AIDS (Quinn, Glasser, & Cannon, 1988; United States Congress Office of Technology Assessment, 1991b).

The most serious of the sexually transmitted diseases is HIV infection (AIDS). Because it takes a number of years between HIV infection and the onset of AIDS, most of the young adults who currently have AIDS acquired HIV infection during adolescence (United States Congress Office of Technology Assessment, 1991b: 257). Yet the actual rate of HIV infection among adolescents is very difficult to discern. It is known, however, that in 1988 AIDS was the sixth leading cause of death for 15- to 24-year olds (Kilbourne, Buehler, & Rogers, 1990; Kipke & Hein, 1990; Novello, 1988). Estimates are that 2 of every 1,000 college students are infected with HIV (Kipke & Hein, 1990; Leary, 1989).

---

[10]   It is important to point out that barrier methods of contraception only reduce (and do not prevent) the chances of pregnancy and infection (Hsiao, 1986). For those under age 20 who are sexually active, 16% of women who use diaphragms and 14% of women whose partners use condoms are expected to experience a pregnancy during the first 12 months of use. Studies of condom breakage indicate that once in every 140 acts of intercourse condoms can be expected to rupture thus exposing the users to infection and pregnancy (Consumer Reports, 1989). See Sikand and Fisher (1992) for a more complete discussion of the relative effectiveness of barrier contraceptive methods.

In addition to the risk of infection, sexually active adolescents are at risk for an early and usually nonmarital pregnancy. Pregnancy under age 20 carries higher health risks to the teen than for those 20 to 24 years old. These risks include anemia, pregnancy-related hypertension, renal disease, and eclampsia (Combs-Orme, 1993). They are due in large part to adolescents' poor use of health care resources and the fact that more frequently than not this is their first pregnancy[11] (Combs-Orme, 1993; McArney & Greydanus, 1988).

As Figure1.7 illustrates, in 1987 adolescent sexual activity resulted in approximately one million adolescent pregnancies, nearly half a million births to adolescents, and more than 410,000 abortions to teenagers (Alan Guttmacher Institute, 1989). By 1990, the number of births to adolescents rose to 533,483. Sixty-eight percent of these births were to unmarried mothers (Moore, Snyder, & Halla, 1993).

It is important to point out that the fathers involved in most of these school-aged pregnancies are generally a few years older than the young mothers; often they are adults. According to a study of all marital and extramarital births to teens aged 11 to 18 in California during 1990, for instance, 85% of the fathers were adults[12] (Males, 1993a). The same study indicates that often the age gap is significant; the partners of those experiencing a pregnancy while they were under 12 years of age were on average 9.8 years older than the young mother (Males, 1993a).

A number of physiological consequences for these young women are associated both with giving birth and with abortion. Medical complications of giving birth include pregnancy-induced hypertension, anemia, depression, hemorrhage, and sepsis.[13] According to one study of urban births to mothers under 20, complications of labor and delivery occurred frequently; more than one third of the young women experienced such complications (Hardy, 1991). Current estimates of maternal death during or shortly following delivery are 6.8 in every 100,000 births to those under the age of 20[14] (National Center for Health Statistics, 1993: 127).

---

[11]   These illnesses are more common among primiparous women (Combs-Orne, 1993).

[12]   This study involved analysis of over 45,000 births in California. Similar results are described, however, from other states as well (Males, 1993a).

[13]   A serious infection characterized by the presence of pus-forming pathogenic organisms, or their toxins in the blood and tissues (Hensyl, 1990).

[14]   In comparison, the maternal mortality rate for those age 20 to 29 was 5.9 per 100,000 live births during 1991 (National Center for Health Statistics, 1993: 127).

FIGURE 1.7:   Pregnancy Outcomes for Adolescents in 1983 (N =1,051,370)

Fetal Deaths (13%)

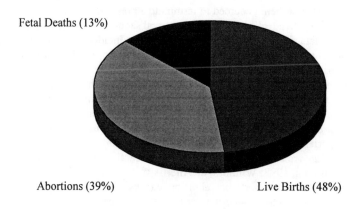

Abortions (39%)   Live Births (48%)

SOURCE: Adapted from Pittman & Adams, 1988 *Teenage Pregnancy, An Advocate's Guide to the Numbers*, Children's Defense Fund, Table 1.2: 10.

Those who terminate their pregnancies are subject to medical complications including infertility, and difficulties with subsequent pregnancies such as having an incompetent cervix, subsequent miscarriage, and premature birth, but these difficulties have not been found to be more common for young women than among the general population of women who give birth (Koop, 1992). The relative medical risk of abortions increases with the duration of the pregnancy; maternal physical complications are more serious for "second and third trimester abortions when hemorrhage, bowel injury, or a perforated uterus may occur" (Koop, 1992: 739). The reported maternal mortality rate associated with legal abortions is annually less than one death per 100,000 procedures (Henshaw, 1990; Koonin, Smith, Ramick, & Lawson, 1992).

Despite extensive discussion of the issue, the evidence concerning the likelihood of a negative psychological impact of abortion on the young

158,366

mother remains inconclusive.[15] In part, because of their methodological weaknesses, many studies are unable to distinguish any negative psychological effects on the mother from those of bringing her baby to term[16] (Koop, 1992: 733; Posavac & Miller, 1990). While substantial evidence exists that being coerced to terminate a pregnancy increases the likelihood of negative feelings of grief, anger, and sadness on the part of the mother, the data do not clearly indicate the likely incidence of adverse psychological reactions to abortion (Russo, 1992; Sheeran, 1987; Wilmoth, 1992). Most existing studies are relatively short term, do not control for pre-pregnancy differences among those who terminate and those who bring the baby to term, are based on anecdotal evidence or other unrepresentative samples, and use measures of unknown reliability and validity (Wilmoth, de Alteriis, & Bussell, 1992). While most researchers agree that some women experience negative psychological reactions following abortions, it is the *prevalence* and likely severity of those reactions which are hotly debated (Wilmoth, 1992; Wilmoth, de Alteriis, & Bussell, 1992).

Many researchers assert that abortion carries with it "significant" psychological risk to the mother (Barard, 1990; De Verber, Ajzenstat, & Chisholm, 1991; Posavac & Miller, 1990; Speckhard & Rue, 1992; Vaughan, 1990).   Speckhard and Rue (1992) view abortion as a psychosocial stressor and its associated negative reactions as a variant of Post-Traumatic Stress Disorder. Their research suggests that Post-Abortion Syndrome is a series of negative reactions to the abortion and may develop years after the termination.[17]

---

[15]   In his report to the President, then Surgeon General of the United States, C. Everett Koop also noted that the data were inconclusive on this point. He wrote, "...there are almost 250 studies reported in the scientific literature which deal with the psychological aspects of abortion. All of these studies were reviewed and the more significant studies were evaluated by staff in several of the Agencies of the Public Health Service against appropriate criteria and were found to be flawed methodologically. In their view and mine, the data do not support the premise that abortion does or does not cause or contribute to psychosocial problems. Anecdotal reports abound on both sides. However, individual cases cannot be used to reach scientifically sound conclusions" (Koop, 1992: 733).

[16]   Both pregnancy and abortion are known to be associated with at least slight incidences of adverse mental health effects (Koop, 1992; Posavac & Miller, 1990).

[17]   Speckhard and Rue (1992: 105) state that the four basic components of Post-Abortion Stress Disorder are: "(1) exposure to or participation in an abortion experience, i.e., the intentional destruction of one's unborn child, which is

It is clear that most adolescents who experience a nonmarital, unexpected, and generally unwanted pregnancy[18] are also subject to the potentially adverse social consequences of either bearing and subsequently parenting their baby or choosing to abort the baby and subsequently dealing with their role in the child's death.[19]   The social consequences of childbearing as an adolescent include long term negative socioeconomic effects, reduced educational attainment and employability (Ahn, 1994; Hayes, 1987; Hofferth & Hayes, 1987; Voydanoff & Donnelly, 1990). Teenage childbearing is also tied to early marriage which has a subsequent higher risk of divorce. The children of adolescents are, in turn, more likely than those whose mothers are over 20 at the time of their birth to be neglected and abused, have difficulty in school, have health problems, to initiate sexual activity at younger ages, and to become adolescent parents themselves (Althaus, 1994; Russo, 1992).

Nutrition and Fitness

The nutritional and fitness needs of many adolescents in the United States are not being met. At one extreme, some suffer from low levels of physical activity and obesity, while others have nutritional deficiencies or eating disorders (United States Congress Office of Technology Assessment, 1991b). According to the 1985 National Children and Youth Fitness Study II, more than 40% of 5th through 12th graders failed to engage in large-

---

perceived as traumatic and beyond the range of usual human experience; (2) uncontrolled negative reexperiencing of the abortion death event, e.g., flash-backs, nightmares, grief, and anniversary reactions; (3) unsuccessful attempts to avoid or deny abortion recollections and emotional pain, which result in reduced responsiveness to others and one's environment; and (4) experiencing associated symptoms not present before the abortion, including guilt about surviving."

[18]   Adler (1992) argues that there are a number of important dimensions or types of pregnancies. Variations in the context of pregnancies include dimensions of wantedness, planning, and intention as well as variations in the mother's age and marital status.

[19]   Another option for adolescents is bearing the child and subsequently releasing the baby for adoption. While this option is chosen by relatively few adolescents--2 to 4%--some data indicate that releasing for adoption reduces some of the adverse socioeconomic impact of adolescent parenthood without causing negative psychological consequences among the mothers (Bachrach, London, & Stolley, 1990; Donnelly & Voydanoff, 1993; McLaughlin, Winges, & Manninen, 1988, 1989; Moore, 1988).

muscle physical activity for at least 20 minutes three times a week throughout the year. The findings of this study indicate that approximately one third of American adolescents are not physically active enough for aerobic benefit (McGinnis, 1987; Ross & Gilbert, 1985). Griesemer and Hough (1993) report only 37% of ninth through twelfth graders participate in health promoting physical activity.[20]

According to one poll, only 21 percent of teens eat three meals a day--and many of those meals are low in nutrients like iron and calcium while they are high in fat (Broihier, 1993). Approximately one fifth of U. S. adolescents are overweight or obese (Bandini, 1992; United States Congress Office of Technology Assessment, 1991b). These adolescents run an increased risk of hypertension, high blood cholesterol, coronary artery disease, various type of orthopedic problems, certain cancers, and gall bladder disease (Bandini, 1992; Dietz, Gross, & Kirkpatrick, 1982; Must, Jacques, & Dallal, 1992). They have a low functional capacity and frequently a low self-concept (Bruch, 1975; Neumann & Jenks, 1992).

A smaller proportion of teenagers have eating disorders which cause them to be seriously underweight. These disorders (anorexia nervosa and bulimia)[21] are estimated to affect about 2.5% of the 15- to 19-year olds. Researchers estimate that at least 0.5% of adolescent and young adult women meet the diagnostic criteria for anorexia nervosa and 1-3% are diagnosed with bulimia nervosa (Fisher, 1992). About half of those with anorexia nervosa also experience bulimia (Coupey, 1992). While most of the young people with these eating disorders are female, about 5 to 10% of bulimic or anorexic adolescents are males (Coupey, 1992; Fisher, 1992).

Each of these disorders is accompanied by serious health problems and in some cases death[22] (Comerci, 1992; Fisher, 1992; Kaplan & Woodside, 1987; United States Congress Office of Technology Assessment, 1991b). Adolescents with bulimia nervosa who abuse laxatives, diuretics, or drink

---

[20] The authors cite the national 1990 Youth Risk Behavior Survey for this estimate (Griesemer & Hough, 1993: 62).

[21] Anorexia nervosa and bulimia are distinct conditions. The diagnostic criteria for anorexia nervosa include the refusal to maintain normal body weight through self-starvation, an intense fear of becoming fat, and a disturbed sense of one's own body. Bulimia entails a morbid hunger--generally manifested as episodic binge eating--and a feeling of lack of control over eating (Comerci, 1992).

[22] Estimates of mortality rates for anorexia and bulimia range from 0 to 22%. Most studies report a mortality rate of approximately 4% for these disorders (Fisher, 1992).

inordinate quantities of water, often experience severe electrolyte abnormalities which may be life-threatening. Gastrointestinal disorders arising from these eating disorders may involve the esophagus, intestines, stomach, kidneys and pancreas (Crisp, 1985; Cuellar & Van Thiel, 1986; Kaplan, 1990). Those who suffer from these disorders often have cardiovascular problems (Comerci, 1992; Kaplan, 1990). Their hearts often decrease in size and functioning; many of the deaths attributable to these eating disorders are heart-related.

Young people who are bulimic or anorexic may also experience the cognitive consequences of starvation such as lethargy, inability to concentrate, irritability, apathy, and sometimes even psychotic disorders (Fisher, 1992; Kaplan & Woodside, 1987). Many adolescents having these disturbed eating habits also experience depression or severe mood swings. In some cases this depression precipitates a suicide or a suicide attempt. The most common cause of death among those suffering from both anorexia or bulimia is suicide (Comerci, 1992; Fisher, 1992; Shisslak, Craso, & Neal, 1990).

Suicide

Suicide accounts for approximately 10% of the deaths of 10- to 19-year-olds (United States Congress Office of Technology Assessment, 1991b). The death rate attributable to suicide is 16 per 100,000 15- to 19-year-olds. Suicide consistently ranks as the second or third leading cause of death among adolescents and has nearly tripled since 1950 (Brent, Perper, Allman, Moritz, Wartella, & Zelenak, 1991; Fingerhut & Kleinman, 1989; Tishler, 1992; Lee, 1993; Vaughan & Litt, 1990d). One study indicates that 12% of all emergency room visits are caused by adolescent suicide attempts (Rauenhorst, 1972). A review of recent studies of adolescent suicide reveals that between 3.5% and 11% of American teens will attempt to kill themselves during their high school years (Lewinsohn, Rohde, & Seeley, 1994; Setterberg, 1992).

Many of the young people who commit suicide--though certainly not all--are experiencing major depression. Some experience other psychopathies such as conduct, affective, or impulse disorders or schizophrenia (Brent, Perper, Goldstein, Kolko, Allen, Allman, & Zelenak, 1988; Hodgman, 1990; Lewinsohn, Rohde, & Seeley, 1994; Kachur, Potter, Powell, & Rosenberg, 1995; Setterberg, 1992). Very often, alcohol consumption is related to suicide; more than half of young suicide victims have significant blood alcohol levels when they die (Hodgman, 1990). Some research suggests that suicide is more frequent among adolescents who are chronically or acutely ill. While it is not known how many seriously ill youths die of suicide but are considered victims of their chronic illness, some studies show, for example, a "disconcerting frequency" of such deaths in patients on dialysis (Hodgman, 1990: 92). Gay and lesbian adolescents, those who are members of rigid, inflexible families, those who have recently experienced the death of other family members by violence, suicide, or accident, those who are members of families who have recently or repeatedly moved, and those who have been physically or sexually abused are more likely than others to commit (or attempt to commit) suicide (Coupey, 1989; Harrington & Dubowitz, 1995; Henry, Stephenson, Hanson, & Hargett, 1993; Hodgman, 1990; U. S. Congress, Office of Technology Assessment, 1991c).

Violence

Interpersonal violence is another major cause of death and disability in the United States (Donnerstein, & Linz, 1995; Hechinger, 1992). In 1990, 12 percent of all homicide victims (2,348) were under 20 years of age (Flanagan & Maguire, 1992). Homicide is now the second leading cause of death among adolescents (Spivak, 1991). Perhaps because of the prevalence and availability of firearms,[23] the homicide rate among U.S. adolescents is higher than in any other country[24] (Cohall & Cohall, 1995; Fingerhut & Kleinman, 1990; Price, Desmond, & Smith, 1991). Weapons and their concomitant violence are prevalent in many high schools in this country (Ginsberg & Loffredo, 1993). High-school-aged teens committed more than 7000 homicides with guns and 4600 without the use of firearms during the 1980s (Flanagan & Maguire, 1992).

Intentional, interpersonal violence also accounts for many serious injuries among adolescents. For each homicide, there are as many as 100 non-fatal injuries serious enough to warrant care by a physician. The vast majority of the victims of violence by adolescents are other adolescents (United States Department of Justice, 1992). Violence by adolescents against a brother or sister is also extremely common. Straus and Gelles

---

[23]   As of 1992, it was estimated that there are 67 million handguns in the United States (Chafee, 1992).

[24]   Data presented by Sloan and his co-authors comparing hand-gun regulations, crime, assaults, and homicides in Seattle with those of Vancouver indicate a clear association between handgun control and less handgun violence. Rates of simple assault and homicide without the use of a handgun were similar in Vancouver and Seattle but assault with the use of a firearm was 7.7 times higher and firearm homicide was about 5 times more frequent in Seattle than in Vancouver which has strict regulations on handgun ownership (Sloan, Kellermann, Reary, Ferris Koepsell, Rivara, Rice, Grary, & LoGerfo, 1988).

(1992: 97) point out that more than one third of 15- to 17-year-olds in the U.S. (approximately four million young people) seriously assault a sibling over the course of a year.[25]

Violence in the form of abuse or neglect by a parent or other family member is very common among adolescents. According to data from the National Center on Child Abuse and Neglect, about 26 of every 1,000 12- to 17-year olds have been victims of this type of violence (Gans, Blyth, Elster, & Gaveras, 1990; National Center on Child Abuse and Neglect, 1988). By most calculations, adolescents are more likely to be sexually and physically abused than any other age group of children (American Medical Association Council on Scientific Affairs, 1993; Gans, Blyth, Elster, & Gaveras, 1990: 21; National Center on Child Abuse and Neglect, 1988; Oreskovich & Bensel, 1991). Figure 1.8 points out that the older adolescents are especially likely to suffer neglect, and that 30 out of every 1000 adolescents have experienced some form of maltreatment.

In addition to the immediate physical problems associated with abuse and neglect, this type of violence against young people has a number of significant implications for mental health and health-compromising behavior during adolescence (Harrington & Dubowitz, 1995). A long list of negative health conditions has been tied to experiencing physical and sexual abuse. Chronic symptoms such as headaches, dizziness, sleeping and eating disorders, depression, anxiety, suicidal ideation, difficulties in school, truancy, and running away from home, as well as sexually transmitted diseases and pregnancy, are associated with abuse among adolescents (American Medical Association, Council on Scientific Affairs, 1989, 1993;
National Research Council, 1993; Rimsza & Niggemann, 1982). Other risky behaviors such as substance abuse are tied to physical and sexual abuse; a good deal of research suggests that the risk of drug and alcohol abuse in those with a history of sexual abuse or incest is higher than in the general population (Boyer & Fine, 1992; Coleman, 1982; Finkelhor, 1987; Gelles & Cornell, 1990). A National Institute of Justice study indicates that survivors of childhood abuse and neglect are 53% more likely to be arrested as juveniles and 38% more likely to be arrested as adults (Widom, 1992). Furthermore, there is adequate evidence to suggest that those who are abused as young people will be more likely than others to become abusers

---

[25] For this research "seriously assault" includes behaviors the authors refer to as "severe violence." They include "punching, kicking, biting, and attacking with a weapon" (Straus & Gelles, 1992: 451).

FIGURE 1.8:   Rates of Abuse and Neglect Experienced by Younger
                   and Older Adolescents per 1,000 Adolescents

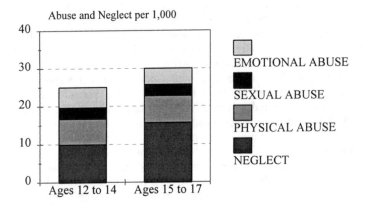

SOURCE: National Center on Child Abuse and Neglect, 1988: 5-1 to 5-45.

of the next generation of children[26] (Gelles & Cornell, 1990; National
Research Council, 1993; Widom, 1992).

Homelessness

Many of the adolescents who are victims of abuse by their parents or
guardians choose to run away from their homes while other adolescents are
forced out of their homes by their parents. In 1988 it was estimated that
nearly half a million young people ran away from home, approximately
112,600 were forced out of their homes or not allowed to come home, and

---

[26] While the strength of the observed relationships between suffering abuse and
      the potential to become an abuser varies greatly from study to study, most
      researchers conclude that a minority of those abused as children will abuse
      their own children.   One commonly quoted study found the rate of
      intergenerational transmission of abuse to be approximately 30 percent
      (Kaufman & Zigler, 1987). Thus being abused increases the risk but does not
      cause one to become abusive (National Research Council, 1993).

about 14,500 were abandoned by their parents (Finkelhor, Sedlak, & Hotaling, 1990). Approximately 1 million adolescents are living on the streets in the United States (American Medical Association Council on Scientific Affairs, 1989a). Homeless adolescents are often malnourished

A homeless teen in Washington, D.C.:

Belinda is eighteen years old, the mother of two young children and homeless. She is staying with her children up the street from Community of Hope at the Pitts Hotel. Belinda feels overwhelmed by the demands of being a single parent and frequently has only a tenuous grip on reality. Sometimes she's afraid she's possessed by the devil, afraid she'll injure her children. During one counseling session with Lois Wagner, Belinda volunteers that she used to dream of a better life, but that she doesn't dream anymore. Lois asks her what kinds of dreams she used to have. Gesturing to indicate the counseling room, simply furnished with a couch, two or three chairs, a stereo, and some pictrures on the walls, Belinda relplies, "Well, I certainly never dreamt I'd live in a beautiful house like this one." Belinda has lost even the ability to imagine anything more that what I would consider substandard housing.

SOURCE: Hilfiker, D., 1994, *Not all of us are saints: A doctor's journey with the poor.*: 112.

and suffering from musculoskeletal, dermatological, gastrointestinal, and genitourinary problems. Homeless youth are more likely than other adolescents to be substance abusers and to have diagnosable psychiatric disorders (American Medical Association, Council on Scientifica Affairs, 1989a). Because these adolescents are unskilled and undereducated, they often turn to prostitution, pornography, and illegal drug trafficking for financial support, thus greatly increasing the risk of sexually transmitted diseases, pregacy, and further victimization (American Medical association council on Scientific Affairs, 1989a; Anderson, Freese, & Pennbridge, 1994).

SOCIODEMOGRAPHIC VARIATIONS

A number of demographic characteristics affect the likelihood that an adolescent will have a serious health problem. These include the more physiological variations of age, sex, and race as well as the social variants such as socioeconomic status, gender, area of residence, and ethnic identification.

Gender and Sex Variations

Some health problems are conditions or behaviors which primarily affect young men; others affect mostly young women. Adolescent males, for example, are more likely to have serious difficulties with acne (United States Congress Office of Technology Assessment, 1991c). Chronic conditions are more common among males than females (Newacheck & Taylor, 1992). They are four times more likely than females to die of suicide, nearly four times as likely to be heavy drinkers, three times more likely to die of homicide, and nearly two-and-a-half times more likely to die of motor vehicle injuries (Fingerhut & Kleinman, 1989; Kachur, Potter, Powell, & Rosenberg, 1995; National Institute on Drug Abuse, 1989b). Nonfatal injuries are also much more frequent for adolescent males than they are for adolescent females (Adams & Hardy, 1989).

Teenage females are uniquely capable of experiencing an early and unexpected pregnancy. They are also about four times more likely than males to be subject to sexual abuse, more likely to be depressed, more likely to be regular smokers, and much more likely to experience eating disorders (Gilchrist, Schinke & Nurius, 1989; National Center on Child Abuse and Neglect, 1988; United States Congress Office of Technology Assessment, 1991b and 1991c; Wauchope & Straus, 1990).

Variations by Age

Adolescents of different ages experience different health risks. Younger adolescents are more likely than those of the older group to suffer from some chronic conditions such as heart disease, asthma, and allergic rhinitis, while acne, orthopedic problems, and bronchitis affect more adolescents between 15- and 18-years-old than those under 15 (United States Congress, Office of Technology Assessment, 1991a: 17; (U.S. Congress, Office of Technology Assessment, 1991b: 159). Older adolescents are subject to higher risk from most of the social morbidities. Adolescents between the ages of 15 and 19 are about five times more likely to die from motor vehicle accidents than are younger adolescents. Older adolescents are also much more likely to die from suicide and homicide than are adolescents under age 15 (Fingerhut & Kleinman, 1989; Kachur, Potter, Powell, & Rosenberg, 1995). Older adolescents are more likely than younger ones to engage in early sexual activity (Hayes, 1987; Voydanoff & Donnelly, 1990). Older adolescents are much more likely than younger teens to be current smokers; they are also more likely to be heavy smokers (Moss, Allen, Giovino, & Mills, 1992; National Center for Health Statistics, 1994). Similarly, the likelihood of using illicit drugs such as marijuana and cocaine increases with the age of the adolescent. For example, the National Center for Health Statistics estimates that in 1991 approximately 4% of the country's youth aged 14 or 15 had used marijuana in the past month while 9% of those aged 16 or 17 used marijuana during the same period (National Center for Health Statistics, 1994: Table 64).

Variations by Income

In the United States, income is generally inversely proportional to health risk and proportional to the services available to address the health needs of adolescents. Indeed, poverty is probably the single most important variable in shaping an adolescent's health and well-being. Poor adolescents are subjected to a host of pathogens and social conditions which are likely to undermine their health.

The principal referred Genene to me because she was so often late to school. The thin, listless, 14-year-old was cleanly dressed when we talked. It seems she lived with her ten-year-old sister and her mother who was a crack-addicted prostitute. Their utilities were often disconnected; it was not unusual for the mother to bring her Johns home. Because there was rarely food or money at home, Genene relied on the school lunch program for most of her nutritional needs.

"I always tell my sister to eat everything they give her at school," the shy ninth-grade student explained, "Lots of times that's all there is. I try to make sure that she has clean clothes and gets on her bus in the morning. Sometimes that means I'm late."

SOURCE: M. Carrick, RN, MS, conversation with the author, June 28, 1996.

As can be seen in Figure 1.9, poverty's impact on the health of adolescents is clear; poorer adolescents are less likely than others to report themselves in excellent health (U.S. Congress, Office of Technology Assessment, 1991c). Adolescents from low-income families are more likely than wealthier teens to have acute or chronic physical conditions--e.g. diseases of the respiratory system or diseases of the musculoskeletal system and connective tissue--that limit their activities (U.S. Congress, Office of Technology Assessment, 1991a; U.S. Congress, Office of Technology Assessment, 1991b; Newacheck, 1989b). Furthermore, rates of diagnosable mental disorders are higher among adolescents from low-income families than among adolescents in higher income brackets (Gans, Blyth, Elster, & Gaveras, 1990; U.S. Congress, Office of Technology Assessment, 1991b; Offer, Ostrov, & Howard, 1991).

FIGURE 1.9:   Percent of U.S. Adolescents Reporting Themselves in Excellent Health by Family Income, 1988.

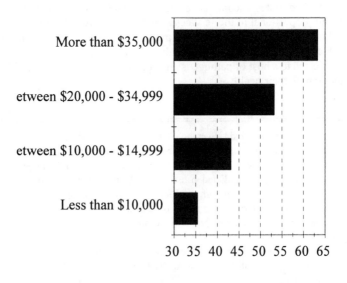

SOURCE: U.S. Congress, Office of Technology Assessment, *Adolescent health-Volume III: Crosscutting issues in the delivery of health and related services,* 1991c: 167 (Table 18-1).

Family income is also a significant predictor of reported physical and mental maltreatment at the hands of others (Dodge, Bates, & Pettit, 1990; Wauchope & Straus, 1990; Straus & Smith, 1992). According to data from the 1988 Incidence Study, the rates of maltreatment are five times higher for children living in families with annual incomes of less than $15,000 than for other children and the rate of neglect among poor children is twelve times higher than among those with higher incomes (Oreskovich & Bensel, 1991, data from the 1988 National Incidence Study). Since poor families often live in neighborhoods where violence and crime are endemic, poor adolescents are much more likely to be the victims of crime. Prothrow-Stith, in her analysis of adolescent violence, points out that middle class adolescents are much less likely than poorer youth to die or to be seriously injured during an assault (1991: 65).

There is also reason to believe that a few adolescent health problems are exacerbated by affluence. According to Wise and Schorr, certain aspects of an affluent environment are associated with negative health outcomes such as drug and alcohol abuse, suicide, motor vehicle accidents, severe narcissism,[27] and some eating disorders (1992: 167-168). These authors speculate that those growing up in wealthy circumstances may be more likely than others to be the subject of unrealistic or destructive parental expectations, have too little experience with delaying gratification, and have relatively easy access to cars, drugs, and alcohol (Wise & Schorr, 1992). Parental influence may be weakened by frequent or prolonged absences and those hired as substitute caretakers (governesses, housekeepers, and boarding school personnel) may be unable or unwilling to provide the consistent and profound caring, nurturance, supervision, and discipline needed for healthy development (Shine, 1992; Wise & Schorr, 1992).

Variations by Area of Residence

Variations in the relative health and well-being of adolescents are also related to where they live. For example, those who live in rural areas are subject to different living conditions than are those in more populated areas. Regional variations also affect patterns of morbidity among adolescents, along with their access to health care delivery systems.

The largest differences between rural and urban morbidity appear to be in the rates of accidental injuries. The higher risk of accidental injury

---

[27] Also called the "silver-spoon syndrome," this complex of symptoms is characterized by an action-orientation, lack of empathy, chronic mild depression, and a low regard for private self (LeBeau, 1988).

among rural youth apparently is closely tied to the use of farm machinery (especially tractors) and to firearm injuries (Paulson, 1990; Rivara, 1985; U.S. Congress, Office of Technological Assessment, 1991c). Drownings are also somewhat more prevalent in rural areas (McManus & Newacheck, 1989; Smith & Brenner, 1995; U.S. Congress, Office of Technological Assessment, 1991c). The rate of death of rural teens due to motor vehicle accidents far exceeds that for adolescents who live in any metropolitan area (Fingerhut, Ingram, & Feldman, 1992a; Walker, Harris, Blum, Schneider, & Resnick, 1990).

When compared with metropolitan teenagers, rural adolescents make fewer visits to physicians each year. The families of rural adolescents often let longer periods of time elapse between visits to their physicians. Perhaps because their ailments are more serious by the time they seek medical treatment, these adolescents are much more likely than those living in urban or suburban areas to be hospitalized (Gans, McManus & Newacheck, 1991; U.S. Congress, Office of Technological Assessment, 1991c).

Inner-city life is associated with its own health risks; violence, threat of violence, and violent crime are more common in inner cities than in suburban or rural areas. Homicide deaths in inner-city areas are much more frequent than in other urban or nonmetropolitan areas. Nearly 28 out of every 100,000 persons 15 to 19 years old in the metropolitan cores were victims of firearm homicide in 1989. Comparable firearm rates in nonmetropolitan areas, fringe, medium, and small metropolitan areas were 2.9, 4.9, 7.5, and 5.7 respectively (Fingerhut, Ingram, & Feldman, 1992a: 49). Nonfirearm homicides, while much less frequent, show a similar distribution across urbanization levels (Fingerhut, Ingram, & Feldman, 1992a: 49).

There are also some regional health differences. Adolescent women in the Southern region of the nation, for instance, are more likely to give birth as teenagers than those in the Northeast and Midwest. Twenty-one percent of all births in Mississippi and approximately 17% of the births in Alabama, Georgia, Kentucky, Louisiana, South Carolina, Tennessee, and West Virginia were to adolescents. In other areas of the country the percent of births to teens was much lower: 7% in Minnesota, about 8% in New Hampshire, North Dakota, and Massachusetts, and about 9% in Connecticut, Iowa, New Jersey, Nebraska, New York, and Iowa (Children's Defense Fund, 1991).

Similarly, poverty--with all its associated health-risks--is not evenly distributed geographically throughout the nation. Figure 1.10 illustrates these regional differences. Notice that the South--the region with the highest teen birth rate--is also the area with the highest poverty rate.

FIGURE 1.10:   Percent of Children Living in Poverty by Region of the Country, 1987

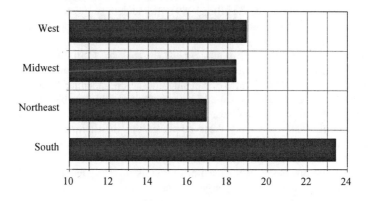

SOURCE: Adapted form Children's Defense Fund, *The State of America's Children, 1991*: 147.

Variations by Race and Ethnic Identity

Health risks also vary markedly by race and ethnic identity among adolescents in this country (Polednak, 1989). Research suggests that Native American teenagers are in poorer health than their White counterparts by almost every measure of health. They are more likely to suffer from hearing impairment, developmental difficulties, obesity, depression, alcoholism, accidents, pneumonia, and dental disease (McShane, 1988; U.S. Congress, Office of Technology Assessment, 1990; Lamarine, 1989). Black adolescent females are more likely than other female teens to suffer from iron-deficiency anemia or obesity (Fitzpatrick, Chacko, & Heald, 1984; Bailey, Ginsburg, Wagner, Neumann & Jenks, 1992; Bailey, Ginsburg, Wagner, Noyes, Christakis, & Dinning, 1982). Sickle-Cell Anemia[28], a condition which worsens significantly during adolescence, is found primarily in children of African American heritage; one in 600 Blacks in the

---

[28]   This disease is caused by an abnormality in the red blood cells which causes them to have a distorted shape. This causes the cells to block small blood vessels often causing damage to various organs and increasing the susceptibility to infections.

U.S. suffers from this disorder and all its accompanying chronic and painful symptoms (Gibbs, 1988a). There is some evidence that Mexican American youth may experience higher rates of obesity and depression than do White adolescents (U.S. Congress, Office of Technology Assessment, 1991c; Mendoza, Martorell, & Castillo, 1989). Some data suggest that indigent Mexican American youth are more likely to test positively for tuberculosis; they are also more likely to have severe acne or eczema problems than are other indigent populations of adolescents (Fitzpatrick, Fujii, Shragg, Rice, Morgan, & Felice, 1990). Recent adolescent immigrants from Indochina have exceptionally high rates of parasitic infestations, anemia, tuberculosis, hepatitis B, and developmental delays. Goiters, skin problems, visual defects, hearing loss, psychosomatic illness, and idiopathic scoliosis are also more common among these ethnic groups than among most other ethnic or racial groups in this country (Fitzpatrick, Johnson, Shragg, & Felice, 1987).

The whole range of social morbidities is directly tied to the ethnic identity of the teens. White youths are nearly three times more likely to die of motor vehicle accidents and more than twice as likely to die of suicide than Black teenagers. Conversely, Black 15- to 19-year old males are ten times more likely to be victims of homicide than are White male adolescents of the same ages; they are also more likely to contract tuberculosis and to display symptoms of hypertension (Gibbs, 1988b). Unlike for other racial and ethnic groups, homicide is the leading cause of death for Black females aged 15 to 19 (Fingerhut & Kleinman, 1989; National Center for Health Statistics, Advance Data, 1993). Native American adolescents experience death from accidental injury at twice the rate of other teens and they have exceptionally high suicide rates as well (Kachur, Potter, Powell, & Rosenberg, 1995; U.S. Congress, Office of Technology Assessment, 1991c). As still another indication that violence is not evenly distributed throughout the society, Black children are abused at significantly higher rates than are White children (Straus & Smith, 1992).

Because some nonwhite adolescents initiate sexual activity at earlier ages than do White adolescents, there are major racial and ethnic differences in pregnancy, abortion, and birth rates among teenage women (Voydanoff & Donnelly, 1990; Forste & Tienda, 1992). One in 20 White female adolescents gave birth in 1987 while one in 11 Latinas gave birth (Children's Defense Fund, 1990). Asian American adolescents have lower pregnancy rates than do White or other nonwhite adolescents (U.S. Congress, Office of Technology Assessment, 1991c). In 1991 there were 27 births per 1000 Asian American adolescent females, 53 per 1000 Euro-American girls, and 116 per 1000 African American adolescent females (Children's Defense Fund, 1994). Sexually transmitted disease rates (including those for HIV infection) are also higher for Black adolescents

(Aral, Schaffer, Mosher, & Cates, 1988; Braverman, 1996; Kulig, 1996; U.S. Congress, Office of Technology Assessment, 1991).

Substance use and abuse also vary among adolescents of different racial and ethnic groups. A significantly higher percentage of White youth than nonwhite adolescents report smoking cigarettes. Researchers have found that Native American teens "begin abusing various substances at younger ages than do other racial and ethnic groups and are more likely to use multiple drugs in combination" (Gans, Blyth, Elster, & Gaveras, 1990: 58; U.S. Congress, Office of Technology Assessment, 1990). Latino youth are more likely than non-Latino Black or White adolescents to have used cocaine (*National Household Survey on Drug Abuse: Population Estimates 1988*, 1989). Even among Latinos, however, there are important ethnic variations; Mexican Americans are *more* likely than Puerto Ricans and Cuban Americans to have ever tried marijuana and *less* likely than Puerto Ricans and Cuban Americans to have ever used cocaine (Gans, Blyth, Elster, & Gaveras, 1990: 58; National Institute on Drug Abuse, 1987).

Interrelationships Among Adolescents' Sociodemographic Characteristics

These variables generally do not influence the health of adolescents in a vacuum; their influence is often indirect and tangled up with a host of other factors. Being a White adolescent does not *cause* one to smoke cigarettes but increases the likelihood that tobacco is regularly used by one's parents and increases the likelihood that there will be funds available to buy it. Being poor does not *make* a teen become obese but it *limits* the adolescent's food choices and is likely to be associated with having a poorly educated parent who does not understand the intricacies of good nutrition. Being African American does not necessarily mean that one will be exposed to the rampant violence of the inner-city but it does influence one's chances of experiencing poverty. Being poor makes it more likely that the family's housing opportunities are limited to less-than-desirable neighborhoods. Jewelle Taylor Gibbs, in her analysis of the health of young Black males in this country, points out that poor Black youth are more likely than most others to live in substandard housing--housing which makes them more vulnerable to:

> . . . chronic respiratory problems from insufficient heat, infestation from lice and other vermin, bites from rats and insects, and lead poisoning from peeling paint. Because they are often reared in single-parent families and may not receive consistent supervision, they are also prone to more household and street accidents, traumas, and other noxious events. (Gibbs,

1988a: 222)

Clearly, being poor makes it more unlikely that one's parents will have completed a college education, found employment, and moved to an area that provides cultural expectations and opportunities that support their adolescents' decisions to postpone early sexual activity. Poor families are more likely than those with more resources to experience unemployment and its associated stresses; families undergoing a stress such as unemployment are less likely to find the resources and energy to negotiate the maze of service delivery systems--often leaving medical treatment until the conditions have become serious enough to warrant hospitalization. The socio-demographic factors that are tied to the health of American teens are interrelated. These social factors have overlapping and sometimes counter-balancing influences on the lives of young people.

INTERRELATED HEALTH PROBLEMS

Health problems occur in a societal context that includes each of these sociodemographic factors as well as the presence of weak labor markets, poor schools, unsafe and deteriorated neighborhoods, the drug culture and violence, family disorganization, and the lack of access to health and social services (Morrill & Gerry, 1990). In addition, as these conditions and problems accumulate, their effects on families and individuals compound and intensify. Studies cited by Lisbeth Schorr (1988) indicate, for example, that low-birth-weight babies experience later cognitive and social impairment only under unfavorable environmental circumstances such as low income and living in a deteriorated neighborhood. Other research indicates that child abuse is more likely when the family is experiencing stressors such as unemployment, alcoholism, or drug addiction (Willging, Bower, & Cotton, 1992).

Therefore, not even all adolescents with a given sociodemographic profile are equally likely to suffer from the same health problems. Often it is the specific overlap or pattern of behaviors that is likely to compromise the adolescents' health and social competence. Nevertheless, teens who suffer from one health problem are likely to suffer from related difficulties. For example, many of the biomedical conditions tend to exacerbate some mental health problems (Friedman & Weiner, 1993). Similarly, the social morbidities affecting adolescents are closely tied to the mental and physical condition of the adolescents.

Clustering of Health-Compromising Behaviors

Teens who often engage in one health-compromising behavior are likely candidates for further risk-taking behavior. Smoking as an adolescent, for example, is correlated with the use of illicit drugs; depression is tied to substance abuse; heavy substance abuse is associated with early sexual activity; and, early sexual activity is tied to early pregnancy, substance abuse, and the consumption of alcohol (Dryfoos, 1990b; U.S. Congress, Office of Technology Assessment, 1991b). Other studies also indicate that several problem behaviors among adolescents are intercorrelated, including problem drinking, illicit drug use, delinquent behavior, dropping out of school, and early sexual activity and pregnancy (Donovan & Jessor, 1985; Klitsch, 1994b; Mott & Haurin, 1988; Yamaguchi & Kandel, 1987; Vanderschmidt, Lang, Knight-Williams, & Vanderschmidt, 1993). Recent

Clustering of problems:

Though she is nicknamed "Heaven," she seemed to be experiencing something closer to "Hell" when she came to our counseling center. Her story is typical of the young women I have counseled. Instead of teens having separate problems--like an eating disorder or an unexpected pregnancy--multiple traumas seem to be mixed together and sometimes spew forth from one event--like a vine with long roots. Each time you pull, you uncover even more.

Heaven was sexually abused as a young child by her father precipitating her parents' divorce. As a young adolescent she was raped at gun-point by an older man. Then the year she turned sixteen her father died and she was sexually abused by her brother. By the time she came to see me, Heaven had attempted suicide three times, weighed 90 pounds, was bulimic and terribly depressed.

Happily, Heaven is healing now. She continues to fight "feeling fat" but is maintaining a healthy weight and understands the relationship between the past sexual traumas and her feelings of worthlessness, subsequent suicidal actions, bulimia, and severe depression.

SOURCE: Linda Mercuri, RN, MS, LPC, Womanline of Dayton, Inc., Dayton, OH, letter to Joan McGuinness Wagner, June 14, 1995.

data based on 1,168 students from one study of younger adolescents attending middle school in a small city in the midwest indicate that 23% were absent 25% or more of the time (45 or more days) during the 1988-1989 school year. These "chronically absent" students were three times as likely to be sexually active, four times as likely to have been emotionally abused or neglected, six times as likely to use alcohol, and seven times as likely to use marijuana as students who were absent less than 45 days during the school year (New Futures/Community Connections, 1989). Another recent study found that pregnant teenagers are at higher than expected risk for substance use, sexual and physical abuse, domestic violence, and suicidal thoughts and actions (Bayatour, Wells, & Holford, 1992). Homeless and runaway adolescent girls are more likely than other adolescents to be sexually active, to become pregnant and give birth; most (62%) choose to keep their child rather than abort the baby or release for adoption (Ravoira & Cherry, 1992).

The Clustering of Health Problems by Family

Adolescents' health problems also cluster by families. Problematic family relationships have impacts upon the adolescent's health and social competence. Patterson, DeBaryshe, and Ramsey (1989), for example, suggest that poor parental discipline and monitoring can start a process resulting in health-compromising behaviors such as delinquency and antisocial behavior. They propose that poor parental discipline and monitoring leads to behavior problems among adolescents which in turn lead to rejection by normal peers and academic failure. This is followed by the commitment to friendships with those who more often participate in antisocial activities and delinquent behaviors. Poor parental discipline and monitoring are associated with low family income and low levels of parental education. Similarly, family stressors such as unemployment, divorce, and death are tied to parenting quality. In some cases parents' inability to maintain quality discipline in their households stems from deficiencies of their own childhoods; antisocial behavior and poor family management are often passed on from one generation to another.

The reverse is also true: adolescents' problems affect other family members and the stability and quality of family relationships. Just as alcohol abuse is more likely among adolescents in families with alcohol-abusing adults, adolescents who are combative, depressed, or experience an early pregnancy may "cause" a dramatic increase in the stress experienced by other family members.

Within a single family there may also be a pattern of intergenerational interrelated health problems which emerge at specific life-cycle stages of the family members. Problems occurring early in life, if untreated, tend to be carried into and often exacerbated in later stages of life--often during adolescence. For example, untreated vision problems contribute to school problems over a period of years. Those who are unable to move through adolescence successfully in terms of schooling and job training find it difficult to become self-sufficient in adulthood. Often these adolescents and young adults bear children that they are unable to support and raise adequately, thus leading to similar problems in the next generation. In some situations, problems begin before birth. Adolescent mothers are less likely to receive prenatal care and their children are more likely to be born prematurely and to have low birth weights than children of older women. Children born to adolescent mothers (especially poor and unmarried mothers) also experience other difficulties as they grow and develop. These include physical problems, lower educational achievement, mild behavior disorders, antisocial behavior, maltreatment, and the likelihood of repeating the whole process by becoming adolescent parents (Voydanoff & Donnelly, 1990).

A list of problems of such magnitude and complexity can be daunting, leaving one wondering if any proposed solutions can have much of an effect. If a comprehensive approach to adolescent health care requires not just treating medical conditions but also addressing some of the most entrenched and intractable problems society faces, is it possible to make practical suggestions about where to begin? Attempting to avoid the ineffective extremes of discouragement and inaction on the one hand and vacuous platitudes without practical consequence on the other, this report posits the existence of a middle ground. It looks to Roman Catholic theology, especially to its social teaching, for a vision of the human person existing both individually and in community. This theoretical theological basis also has practical implications for developing a plan to deliver adolescent health care.

CHAPTER 2

THE SOCIAL CONTEXT OF ADOLESCENT HEALTH

Attitudes and behaviors concerning health and illness are rooted in the culture of the surrounding society (Fabrega, 1981; Gesler, 1991). A patient's understanding of a medical condition can cause and shape symptoms as well as profoundly influence their remission[29] (Press, 1982). The accepted understandings about health and illness are influenced by available technologies, moral evaluations, scientific paradigms, language systems, and the health care delivery system; the experience of health and illness is defined by the adolescent's social and cultural surroundings.

Cultural anthropologists are careful to point out that experiences of health and illness are regularly influenced by their cultural context. The symptoms a patient chooses to report to a physician, for instance, are the ones the sufferer thinks are relevant to the condition; often they include some which the doctor will not find important or they exclude others which the patient has attributed to some other source. Similarly, the patient's understanding of his or her condition and treatment--a symbolic and cultural phenomenon--is tied to the images and reputations of both the malady and its remedy (Press, 1982). Mainstream Americans as well as ethnic minorities "*always* clothe their diseases in symbolic dress, and are *always* susceptible to symbolic stimuli--both as cause and as aid to cure"

---

[29] Irwin Press (1982: 180-181) explains that such an effect is understandable even within biomedical models of medicine since symbolic phenomena affect the brain and the brain is known to have the ability to stimulate production of chemicals and other physiological reactions in the body. Such brain responses sometimes help to reduce pain, lower blood pressure, reduce the rate of malignant growths, and stabilize heart beats.

(emphasis in the original {Press, 1982: 181}).

The meaning and experience of health and illness are inherently variable. Cultural standards for what is "healthy" and "unhealthy" have changed drastically over time and they vary from one culture to another. Early in this century, for instance, prominent physicians considered college education an unhealthy strain on young women's brains but few recognized cigarette smoking as harmful (Macionis, 1995: 538). Similarly, in some cultures the "cause" of illness is a disruption in the proper balance of certain bodily fluids; others point to what most Americans would consider supernatural causes and cures[30] (Fabrega, 1981; Gesler, 1991; Press, 1982). Some people with cultural ties to Colombia believe that certain days are better than others for healing; some people of Mexican-American heritage believe that an emotional shock or a severe fright causes certain diseases (Press, 1982).

The importance of the specific cultural conditions on some health-compromising conditions cannot be underestimated. All people--adults as well as adolescents--judge their own health by comparing their condition with that of those around them (Macionis, 1995). Adolescents believe themselves to be healthy when the maladies they can see in themselves are no different from those of their friends. Whether or not young persons believe themselves to be healthy stems in part from their culturally-informed expectations. Some years ago, for instance, "yaws, a contagious skin disease, was so common in tropical Africa that societies there considered it normal" (Macionis, 1995: 538). American culture similarly shapes many of adolescents' expectations and definitions of health. It is difficult to imagine, for example, that anorexia nervosa could be understood outside the context of a culture typically portraying the slim, youthful body as healthy and beautiful (Schaeffer & Lamm, 1992).

If the resources of Catholic social and moral teaching are going to be applied credibly to the needs of adolescent health, all the factors affecting that health need to be taken into account. Like their other behaviors and attitudes, adolescents model their health-impacting behaviors on those of the people they see and know. Some learn these behaviors from the general culture, some from their friends, and some from teachers. Two very important sources of health information, behaviors, and attitudes are discussed here: the adolescents' families and the mass media.

---

[30] The cultural systems included are some groups living in India, Pakistan, Bangladesh, China; some of those living in the areas of Europe where humoral medicine is practiced; some groups of Native Americans; and some areas with concentrated Islamic populations. For a more complete discussion of these "traditional" explanations of health and illness see Gesler, 1991.

ROLE OF THE FAMILY IN HEALTH

The discussion of adolescent health must be grounded in an understanding of the important role which families play in the lives of teenagers. This is especially true in the area of health and health-related behaviors, in which research seems to support Catholic social teaching's emphasis on considering adolescents as members of families. Research has revealed that the family influences the health of its members in many ways. Illness, especially chronic illness, is strongly influenced by the nature and structure of the family. Health-influencing behaviors are supported or suppressed by the family, while illness and disabilities affect family members' health and functioning in a number of important ways (Consortium of Family Organizations, 1992; Campbell & Treat, 1990; Doherty & Campbell, 1988).

Doherty and Campbell (1988), in their work on families and health, present an interactive model to summarize the many dimensions of the relationships between families and their members' health. This model can be seen in Figure 2.1. As Doherty and Campbell conceive of it, the model implies a temporal sequence as well as continuous interaction between the family system and the health care system.

This model highlights five major components of family/health interaction. Families are perceived to play a pivotal role in promoting healthy behaviors and reducing health-compromising behaviors. They are important in explaining a member's vulnerability to a physical illness or social morbidity. Families are seen to influence the understanding and interpretation of a condition as health-threatening; they are closely tied to the member's chances of seeking and receiving adequate medical treatment. This model also posits that the acute illness of an individual member will precipitate a family response that may have long-lasting repercussions for both the patient and the family. The fifth component of the Doherty and Campbell "Family Health and Illness Cycle" is the understanding that an individual's adaptation to illness and recovery is closely tied to the family's ability to deal with his or her condition and to negotiate service delivery from the health care system. While not specifically designed with adolescents in mind, this model presents one method of organizing an understanding of the multifaceted relationships existing among adolescents, their families, and health care providers (1988).

Families provide a central vehicle for health promotion and risk reduction through their transmission of beliefs and social behaviors. Specific expectations about appropriate behavior and the appropriate responses to a given situation are taught by parents both verbally and through example. What individuals choose to eat for breakfast, do with their spare time, think or worry about, and the number of children they choose to have are all decisions shaped by the patterns they experience in

FIGURE 2.1:   Family Health and Illness Cycle

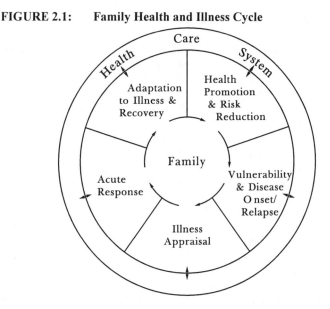

SOURCE: Doherty & Campbell, 1988, *Families and Health,* Figure 1.1:
                  23, reprinted with permission.

their families. Families are a primary source of this complex of learned
behaviors; it is within the context of the family that adolescents learn a
whole range of health-related behaviors (Murphy & Price, 1988;
Schoonmaker, 1983).

The behaviors and attitudes learned within the context of the family
influence the health of adolescents in a number of ways. Those diseases
and conditions that result from learned behaviors are therefore closely tied
to the individual's family situation. Adolescents in families whose diets are
heavy in fat are more likely than those from families who eat more
vegetables to have difficulties with obesity. Adolescents in families that
deal with difficult situations through violence are more likely to turn to
physical violence themselves. Straus and Smith point out, for example, that
children learn to be "violent toward others by being victims of violence at
the hands of their parents" (1990: 255-256). Parents may model drug or
alcohol abuse to their adolescents through their own drug use (Snyder,
1992). Adolescents who smoke are more likely to come from families
where the adults smoke than from non-smoking families (Gilchrist,
Schinke, & Nurius, 1989; Clayton, 1991; Murphy & Price, 1988;
Schoonmaker, 1983). Since a majority of adolescent health problems are
tied directly to lifestyle choices and risky behaviors learned, fostered, or

suppressed by their parents and siblings, the families have a direct and central role in promoting healthy behavior and reducing the risk of illness.

Families contribute to the vulnerability of their adolescents to health problems in complex ways. Many illnesses are in some part genetic; some health conditions or susceptibilities are inherited. Such biological ties to the family explain, however, only a small portion of the impact of the family on an adolescent's chances for health and well-being. Numerous studies have shown that family members, both spouses and offspring, are more likely than unrelated individuals to share the risk factors of chronic health conditions such as hypertension, high cholesterol and obesity (Campbell & Treat, 1990; Barbarin & Tirado, 1985).

Research also indicates that difficulties within the family often have negative health effects on family members. Stress in the family as a result of difficulties such as a divorce, unemployment, the death of a family member, or even the birth of a child, has been documented to have adverse health affects on family members (Campbell & Treat, 1990; Willging, Bower, & Cotton, 1992). The process of divorce, for instance, can create difficulties and demands upon families which ultimately result in illness among the children (Doherty & McCubbin, 1985; Guidubaldi & Cleminshaw, 1985). Stressful life experiences are also tied to an increase in physical violence within families (Straus, 1990). According to some research, "stress has the effect of suppressing the body's immune function and, thus, predisposing individuals to becoming ill" (Consortium of Family Organizations, 1992:9). Other authors have pointed out that problems in families with adolescents may stem from longstanding family issues, disturbed family function, or difficulty in negotiating the transition of the young family member into young adulthood (Snyder, 1992).

The fact that family members share the same or similar access to resources also means that they share many of the same threats to health and chances for well-being. Blue-collar families, for instance, are more likely to experience incidents of physical violence than are members of white-collar families (Wauchope & Straus, 1990). All members of poor families are at substantially higher risk of acute and chronic physical and mental illness than are individuals in wealthier families. All members of poor families are less likely than those with higher incomes to receive timely and adequate health care (Consortium of Family Organizations, 1992).

The family also plays a role in illness appraisal. The adolescent's attitudes toward illness, the experience of pain, and the appropriateness of health care are also directly tied to the attitudes learned within the context of the family. Adolescents will often ask a parent for health care information before turning to a professional. Some families encourage the seeking of treatment, compliance with treatment, and use of prescribed medicines, while others discourage the use of medical services. Families that do not emphasize the importance of self-accountability for even their adult members are unlikely to inspire an attitude of responsibility on the part of their teenagers.

Lastly, family relationships are important in the adaptation to illness and recovery. This is true both of responses to acute health problems and adaptation to chronic illness. The social support derived from close familial ties has a significant positive impact on the physical health and mortality of individual family members (Campbell & Treat, 1990; Doherty & Campbell, 1988). While most research has focused on the role of social support from one's spouse on health outcomes, there is no reason to assume that parental or sibling support would function differently. For example, Hauser and his coauthors (1985) present evidence that the family environment is related to perceived competence and illness adjustment in diabetic and actively ill adolescents.

Different family structures are also tied to variations in relative health. In general, married men are healthier than single men. Furthermore, research indicates that children living in single-parent households are at greater risk for a number of negative health outcomes (Consortium of Family Organizations, 1992; Guidubaldi & Cleminshaw, 1985). According to researchers of the Consortium of Family Organizations, "Marital status and the levels of support available from relatives and friends are the most powerful predictors of health. For the elderly, the presence and number of living children are the most powerful predictors of survival" (1992: 10).

THE INFLUENCE OF MASS MEDIA ON ADOLESCENT HEALTH

Adolescents learn a great deal of information concerning health and illness as well as many of their health-related attitudes and behaviors from both their families and various forms of the mass media. Those they see on television, in the movies, at sporting events, in music videos, those they hear on the radio and CD's, and those they read about in newspapers and magazines each have the potential of influencing the teens' health-related knowledge and behaviors.

Unfortunately, the information and behaviors that teens learn from these sources are often biased, inaccurate, or unhealthy. As Signorielli (1993) points out, television presents to the viewer a slanted perspective on health by minimizing the social context of disease and by emphasizing its biomedical component.

Television characters typically do not get sick because they do not have enough food, or live in substandard or unsanitary housing. Moreover, except in very rare situations, characters do not have to worry about having health insurance or enough money to pay for a hospital stay or a doctor's care (Signorielli, 1993: 26).

In general, physicians are portrayed unrealistically as having unlimited time and resources to devote to individual patients. Death is almost always depicted as the end result of violence rather than of natural causes (Cassata, Skill, & Boadu, 1983; Signorielli, 1993). On television, recovery from an illness appears to be more dependent on the character's role in the program than it is on their health promoting behaviors or even the quality of the medical care they receive; the " 'good' characters are likely to recover and 'bad' characters deserve their fate" (Signorielli, 1993: 18). Indeed, many of the behaviors and attitudes touted by the media closely correspond to those doing so much harm among the adolescent population of the nation: violence, substance abuse, suicide, and nonmarital[31] sexual intercourse.

According to the 1992-1993 Nielsen Report on Television, on average, adolescents spend approximately 22 hours watching television each week[32] (AC Nielsen Company, 1993: 9). During their school years, these teens spend more time watching television than they do in school, in sporting activities, or in church; they spend more time watching television than in any other activity except sleeping (Strasburger, 1986 and 1993).

Given so much time spent watching television, it is reasonable to expect adolescents to be affected by their viewing. There are two major reasons why this causes concern among those interested in the health and well-being of teenagers. First, those involved in heavy television viewing are less likely to spend time in activities which promote healthy growth. Obesity, for example, is associated with heavy television viewing at least in part because of its displacement of exercise (Dietz, 1993; Dietz & Gortmaker, 1993; Strasburger, 1993). Similarly, school performance is lower for those who watch a lot of television than it is for those who do not, perhaps because time spent watching television is not then spent on school

---

[31]   The term 'nonmarital sexual activity' rather than 'premarital sexual activity' is chosen deliberately for two reasons. First, there is ample evidence that adolescents are modeling their behaviors after adults; within the context of our understanding of Catholic moral teaching, all intercourse outside of the commitment of marriage is problematic. Second, much of the sexual activity of non-married persons is not a precursor of marriage.

[32]   Adolescents spend somewhat less time than younger children viewing television, but they are still "quite heavily exposed" (Morgan, 1993: 609; AC Nielsen, 1993).

work or other reading[33] (Morgan, 1993; Strasburger, 1986).

The second major problem with extensive television viewing involves the behaviors and attitudes young people learn from watching television programs and commercials. Research indicates that television exerts its influence on the behavior of young people by shaping the viewers' attitudes concerning what is and what *should be* (Bryant & Rockwell, 1994; Dietz & Strasburger, 1991; Donnerstein & Linz, 1995; Klein, Brown, Childers, Oliveri, Porter & Dykers, 1993; Signorielli, 1993). Strasburger points out that:

> television may offer older children and younger adolescents scripts about gender roles, conflict resolution, and patterns of courtship and sexual gratification that they may be unable to observe anywhere else. Heavy consumers of television may begin to believe that the world is a more violent place than it really is, that violence is an acceptable solution to any problem, or that all conflicts can be easily resolved within a short period of time.   Similarly, if they watch a lot of soap operas, they may overestimate the number of sexually active teenagers and the incidence of extramarital affairs or underestimate the risk of sexually transmitted disease. (1993: 480)

Thus, television programming is able to skew the viewer's understanding of many health-compromising behaviors.   Violence is rampant and glorified, alcohol usage is often presented positively,[34] and nonmarital sexual activity discussed or alluded to often (Atkin, 1993; Brown, Greenberg, & Buerkel-Rothfuss, 1993; Comstock & Strasburger, 1993; Dietz & Strasburger, 1991; Donnerstein & Linz, 1995; Shiffrin, 1993; Signorielli, 1993; Wallack, Grube, Madden, & Breed, 1990). Comstock and Strasburger, for instance, estimate that American teens view at least 1,000 murders, rapes, and aggravated assaults per year while watching television

---

[33]   A close reading of the arguments concerning the reason for this association indicates no clear consensus among researchers. The relationship between poor school performance and heavy television viewing may be (1) an actual result of the viewing, "(2) a process wherein lower performance leads to heavier viewing, (3) a spurious association resulting from third factors, or (4) all of the above, operating simultaneously and perhaps to different degrees for different students" (Morgan, 1993: 618).

[34]   While alcohol is no longer consumed in commercial portrayals, it is frequently ingested during programs. One research project indicates that alcohol appeared in 64% of all prime-time fictional programs and that characters consumed alcohol in half of the studied programs (Wallack, Grube, Madden, & Breed, 1990: 428).

(1993). Firearms appear on T.V. about 9 times per hour during prime-time programs (Strasburger, 1993). Gerbner's analysis of some 4,000 television programs indicates an average of five incidents of violence each hour (1992). He points out that:

> TV is a world in which men outnumber women at least three to one. This male cast makes the world revolve mostly around questions of power. That is why television is so violent: the best, quickest demonstration of power is a show-down that resolves the issue of who can get away with what against whom. (Gerbner, 1992: 9)

Other researchers point out that adolescents view a great number of sexual encounters during their viewing and that the majority of these are between unmarried couples (Brown, Greenberg, & Buerkel-Rothfuss, 1993; Greenberg, 1994). Rarely do these portrayals of nonmarital sexual encounters refer to their all-too-frequent consequences, such as sexually transmitted diseases, pregnancy, and abortion (Brown, Greenberg, & Buerkel-Rothfuss, 1993; Bryant & Rockwell, 1994). Research indicates that adolescents exposed heavily to viewing of prime-time TV depicting sexual intimacy are likely to alter their moral judgment concerning the appropriateness of nonmarital sexual activity[35] (Bryant & Rockwell, 1994).

Television is not the only form of mass media having the ability to influence the health, attitudes, and behaviors of young people. Teenagers spend almost as many hours a day listening to the radio as they do watching T.V. (Klein, Brown, Childers, Oliveri, Porter, & Dykers, 1993). They are frequent viewers of music videos, see movies often, and read many magazines that continually promote a number of health-risking behaviors. Popular music and music videos, for example, are often focused on themes antithetical to the health and well-being of youth. According to Brown, Greenberg, and Buerkel-Rothfuss (1993) about 75% of song lyrics refer to sex and love; many deal explicitly with lust, masturbation, sexual intercourse, and sexual violence (Greenberg, 1994). Drug abuse and alcohol use are often glamorized in popular music; suicide, racism, and more general forms of violence are also common themes (Hendren & Strasburger, 1993).

The favorite magazines of adolescents present a variety of articles

---

[35] This research also indicates that a number of individual and family factors may mitigate any potential unwanted shifts in values that might occur from watching sexually charged television. These include having a well-defined family value system, free and open discussions of issues within the family, and the ability of the teen to critically view the programs (Bryant & Rockwell, 1994: 194)

focusing on sexual intimacy. Some of the publications specialize in sexually explicit information; others simply use sexually-charged images to increase their sales (Brown, Greenberg, & Buerkel-Rothfuss, 1993). Advertisements in these magazines encourage teens' use of cigarettes, alcohol, and diet programs. They also promote body images that are unrealistic for all but the smallest minority of teens (Kilbourne, 1993). Many ads are overtly sexual; a good number use sexual aggression and violence as a tool to promote the featured product. Kilbourne argues that adolescents:

> . . . learn a great deal about sexual attitudes from the mass media and from advertising in particular. Advertising's approach to sex is pornographic: it reduces people to objects and de-emphasizes genuine human contact and individuality. It often directly targets young people. This reduction of sexuality to a dirty joke and of people to objects is the true obscenity of American culture. Although the sexual sell, overt and subliminal, is at fever pitch in most advertising, depictions of sex as an important and profound human activity are notably absent. A sense of joy is also notably absent; the models generally look either hostile or bored. (Kilbourne, 1993: 644)

Findings from a survey of 2760 14- to 16-year olds in urban areas in this country indicate that teens who engaged in more health-compromising behaviors listened to the radio and watched music videos and movies on television more frequently than those who engaged in fewer risky behaviors (Klein, Brown, Childers, Oliveri, Porter, & Dykers, 1993: 24). The health-compromising behaviors considered in this analysis included some of the more common social morbidities: sexual intercourse, consumption of alcohol, and smoking of marijuana or tobacco. While the causal direction of this relationship is unclear,[36] the very existence of the relationship posits clear challenges to those who create, market, and distribute the forms of media involved; to the adolescents who expose themselves to these influences; and to the parents who permit and foster that exposure.

These first two chapters have attempted to lay out the problems that face anyone interested in improving adolescent health. All those involved will want to draw on the best available research. Those who are also committed either personally or professionally to Catholic tradition have an additional set of resources upon which to draw. This is the long history of theological

---

[36]   That is, it may be that adolescents already involved in these social morbidities choose to listen to more "antisocial" media rather than that the "antisocial" media influences these teens to engage in more health-risking behaviors (Klein, Brown, Childers, Oliveri, Porter, & Dykers, 1993).

reflection on the nature of the human person and on the meaning and purpose of life, Before moving on to the issue of health care use and delivery, we turn to a consideration of how those pragmatic concerns can and should be shaped by a Catholic moral and social vision.

CHAPTER 3

REFLECTIONS ON ADOLESCENT HEALTH CARE FROM CATHOLIC MORAL TEACHING

Presupposing that each human person is a dignified individual and an inherently social being, Catholic social teaching draws upon scripture and tradition to express basic principles and to call people to action. It rules out approaches to social, political, and economic concerns that deny the dignity or social nature of the human person, but its prescriptions are intentionally broad-ranging. It leaves room for competent lay persons in the world to make prudent judgments concerning its application to specific problems.

Vatican II's *Pastoral Constitution on the Church in the Modern World* has two main parts: the first deals with human beings, society, the church, and the kingdom of God; the second addresses "Problems of special urgency"--in particular, marriage and the family, culture, economics, politics, and peace. This document calls Catholics to scrutinize the "signs of the times" (Vatican Council II, 1965: #4), and acknowledges the need for continual updating "since it sometimes deals with matters in a constant state of development" (Vatican Council II, 1965: #91). In recent years, the social teaching of the Church has been extended to such areas as ecology and the role of women in church and society.

It is the judgment of this team of researchers that the current crisis in adolescent health care qualifies as what Vatican II called a "problem of special urgency" (Vatican Council II, 1965: #46). As our survey of statistical studies has demonstrated, this crisis has a dramatic impact on the lives of individuals, on families, and on the very fabric of our society.

The purpose of this segment of our study is to draw upon contemporary Catholic teaching to reflect theologically on the *need* to provide health care to adolescents as well as on the *type* and *quality* of that health care.

WHY HEALTH CARE?

The Catholic Church has a long heritage of caring for the health of individuals and in providing health care in institutionalized settings. Jesus as portrayed in the New Testament was himself a healer, who often tied together healing and forgiveness with the coming of the kingdom of God. Jesus frequently told those who had been healed that it was their faith that had healed them. In the parable of the Last Judgment (Matt 25:31-46), Jesus lists caring for the sick among those things that when done for the least of his are done to him. Caring for the sick is one of the traditional corporal works of mercy;[37] its importance to Christians is as old as Christianity. In the *Acts of the Apostles,* the disciples continue Jesus' ministry, which includes not only leadership and teaching, but also the healing of those afflicted with disease or disability.

Healing has continued throughout Christian history as one dimension of carrying on the mission of Jesus. The new Rite for the Anointing of the Sick highlights the connection between the sacrament itself and the traditional importance of care for the afflicted (Catholic Church, 1976: 571-642). The sacrament is no longer restricted to those who are in imminent danger of death, but has been extended to those who are seriously ill or faced with a threatening medical procedure. More important for our considerations, the new rite encourages the presence of family and friends while the sacrament is being administered. The sacrament is thus linked symbolically with the healing that is mediated through the presence of a caring community that prays, visits, helps out, provides treatment, and fosters a loving environment that encourages the one who is ill to regain health.

As demonstrated in our study, many of the ills that face adolescents and their families today are social in nature. Vatican II's *Pastoral Constitution on the Church in the Modern World,* while maintaining that sin ultimately has its roots in individuals, recognized also the long-term and pervasive effects that sin has on social institutions: "When the structure of affairs is flawed by the consequences of sin, human beings, already born with a bent toward evil, find there new inducements to sin, which cannot be overcome without strenuous efforts and the assistance of grace" (Vatican Council II, 1965: #25). The Church is called to address the presence of sin in social structures:

---

[37] The traditional corporal works of mercy are "feeding the hungry, giving drink to the thirsty, clothing the naked, sheltering the homeless, visiting the sick visiting the imprisoned, and burying the dead" (Stravinskas, 1993: 265).

. . . the Church does not only communicate divine life to human beings but in some way casts the reflected light of that life over the entire earth, most of all by its healing and elevating impact on the dignity of the person, by the way in which it strengthens the seams of human society and imbues the everyday activity of people with a deeper meaning and importance. (Vatican Council II, 1965: #40)

Richard A. McCormick, a specialist in Catholic ethics, links health care delivery with the very mission of the Church:

The Church, the extension of Christ's presence, is in the business of spreading the good news. To spread the good news means to do all those things that remind us of who we are. We are reminded of our true worth by being treated in accordance with this dignity. It is axiomatic that we expand and become capable of love by being loved. Hence the Church's proclamation is necessarily action. The Church is in the health care apostolate because it is a most concrete and effective way of communicating to human beings their real worth--that is, the good news. (1984: 20)

McCormick warns, however, that Catholic health care institutions sometimes mirror the very injustices that they should seek to remedy; for example, in the gender, racial, and class make-up of the staff (1984: 76).

Pastoral theologian Robert L. Kinast, drawing upon Vatican II as well as more recent church documents, characterizes the fundamental mission of the church as one of "caring for society" through the role of lay people in the world (1985: 96-115). In imitation of Jesus, such "care" involves precisely the setting free of people from whatever it is that binds them, whether that be physical, emotional, psychological, social, or spiritual; it involves setting them free _for_ more healthful and fruitful lives, more meaningful existence, deeper human relations, a sense of purpose and direction (Kinast, 1990; Clarke: 252-53). This approach matches well with the stance taken in *Christifideles Laici* by John Paul II (1989), who outlines the major spheres of the Christian activity of lay persons in the world as family, work, and society, with a stress on the transformation of social structures in the direction of ever greater justice and solidarity.

Catholics who address critical matters of health care in the world can thus interpret their activity in harmony with Catholic teaching as part of their Christian mission in the world. It is not necessary that such activity in every case be explicitly "Catholic." As expressed in the *Pastoral Constitution on the Church in the Modern World*:

Now, the gifts of the Spirit are diverse: while the Spirit calls some to give clear witness to the desire for a heavenly home and to keep the desire fresh among the human family, the Spirit summons others to dedicate themselves to the earthly service of human beings and to make ready the material of the celestial realm by this ministry of theirs. (Vatican Council II, 1965: #38)

Some witness, therefore, is implicitly "Catholic" by serving human beings in the interest of the kingdom of God and in a manner that is in harmony with Catholic teaching about the dignity of human beings.

WHY ADOLESCENT HEALTH CARE?

Adolescence is something of an ambiguously defined period in human development. Many societies do not recognize anything that resembles adolescence as we know it, and even in our own society the length and meaning of this period has shifted dramatically over the centuries. Adolescence seems to be a cultural creation for the purpose of allowing more time for education prior to full adulthood in our complex society. In the nineteenth century, labor unions lobbied for increased age limits on child labor laws at least in part to lower unemployment and lessen the amount of labor available (Koteskey, 1991: 48).

Adolescence is a time of contradiction. An adolescent has capacities for mature behaviors, and yet is subject to many social limitations on personal freedom and responsibility. Not quite an adult, yet no longer a child, the adolescent receives mixed messages from a society that has plenty of its own uncertainties and even corruptions. Drugs, sex, and material luxuries are presented as glamorous and desirable even as they are forbidden to the adolescent.

Adolescence is an in-between time. It might helpfully be described by a term used by the cultural anthropologist Victor Turner (1969); it is a *liminal* period. A liminal period is a time of change, a time when the normal rules do not apply, a time of shifting from one established pattern to another. A person in the liminal state is "neither here nor there; they are betwixt and between the positions assigned and arrayed by law, custom, convention, ceremonial" (Turner, 1969: 95; Arbuckle, 1986: 442). For example, the "roaring 20's" and the 1960's were liminal periods in U.S. cultural history. Both eras are widely recognized as times when the established social patterns were "loosened" for what turned out to be a time of transition.

Adolescence is itself a period of prolonged transition. Although many adolescents do lead healthy lives, our study demonstrates that for great numbers of adolescents, the teen years are a time filled with risks, accidents, killings, suicide, alcohol, drugs, and promiscuity. Adolescents are a marginalized group in so far as they live on the outskirts of accepted social patterns. Some commentators argue that there exists an adolescent subculture, complete with its own language, symbols, and values (Davies, 1991; Ekstrom, 1986).

In the New Testament, Jesus is portrayed as one who reaches out to those on the margins. Whether it be the Samaritan woman at the well or Zacharias the tax collector, Jesus seeks out those with whom no one else will bother. In contemporary Catholic social teaching, such outreach is symbolized by the concept of the "preferential option for the poor."[38] As discussed by John Paul II in *Centesimus Annus,* the option for the poor

> . . .is not limited to material poverty, since it is well known that there are other forms of poverty, especially in modern society--not only economic, but cultural and spiritual poverty as well. . . In the countries of the West, different forms of poverty are being experienced by groups which live on the margins of society, by the elderly and the sick, by the victims of consumerism. . . Love for others, and in the first place love for the poor, in whom the church sees Christ himself, is made concrete in the promotion of justice. Justice will never be fully attained unless people see in the poor person, who is asking for help in order to survive, not an annoyance or a burden, but an opportunity for showing kindness and a chance for greater enrichment. (John Paul II, Pope, 1991: #57-58)

This study provides ample evidence why adolescents should be considered as among the "poor" as defined in contemporary Catholic social teaching. They are a group in crisis, in whose faces the face of Christ is to be discerned.

WHAT TYPE OF HEALTH CARE?

There is a tendency in some quarters of our society today to view adolescents as individual consumers who need information and resources to make their own decisions about values and behavioral choices. Catholic social teaching views such an approach as only half-right. The adolescent as individual needs to be understood, but so does the adolescent as social being; the adolescent as consumer needs to be balanced by the adolescent as responsible citizen; the adolescent as informed decider must be

---

[38] According to the *Catholic Dictionary* (Stravinskas, 1993: 394), preferential option for the poor is the "apparent favor shown to the poor in the Church's ministry, shown by Christ in the Gospels and particularly expressed in documents since Vatican II."

complemented by the adolescent who is given sound guidance concerning true and false values.

Health care that dispenses information and devices while dispensing with the fuller social and moral context is not in accordance with Catholic teaching. This is not to say, however, that in our pluralistic society Catholics should insist on an explicit presentation of "Catholic" positions on every relevant issue. Such an insistence would severely limit the ability of Catholic health workers and others to engage the critical problems of our times in the places where they exist. What is more important is that there be a significant Catholic presence that does what it can within the context in which it finds itself.

Such an approach is in harmony with traditional Catholic rejection of solutions to social problems that are "utopian" insofar as they idealistically insist that the world become perfect overnight. Such "solutions" have the tendency to replace a difficult situation with one that is even worse. On the other hand, traditional Catholic teaching rejects just as strongly the approaches of those who throw up their hands in despair at the seeming impossibility of the task at hand. Catholic social teaching has promoted instead a realistic and confident hope, one that trusts that God will collaborate with those who work and pray in earnest for a more just and loving society.

Adolescent health care that reflects the principles of Catholic social teaching will manifest certain characteristics. It will:

> show deep respect for the dignity of each individual person as made in the image and likeness of God;
>
> foster authentic human development;
>
> attend to the common good;
>
> affirm the family as the basic unit of a healthy society;
>
> take seriously the option for the poor;
>
> see that problems are addressed on the most appropriate level of society;[39] and,

---

[39] This approach is called the "principle of subsidiarity" among Catholic scholars. It refers to the understanding that social problems are best addressed at the lowest social level possible. If problems can be solved at the family level, they should be; problems which can be addressed in the local community should not be taken to the national level. It underscores the need

uphold a consistent life ethic.

Dignity of the Individual

The most basic of Catholic beliefs is that human beings are the sacred, unique, and clearest reflection of God's love and presence in our world. This sacredness is manifested in all persons regardless of age, sex, race, or economic status. Pope John XXIII addressed not only Catholics but all people of good will when he linked human dignity with the right to health care:

> Any human society, if it is to be well-ordered and productive, must lay down as a foundation this principle, that every human being is a person; that is, each human being is endowed with intelligence and free will. Indeed, precisely because one is a person, one has rights and obligations flowing directly and simultaneously from one's very nature. And as these rights and obligations are universal and inviolable, so they cannot in any way be surrendered. . .
>
> Beginning our discussion of the rights of human beings, we see that every person has the right to life, to bodily integrity, and to the means which are suitable for the proper development of life; these are primarily food, clothing, shelter, rest, medical care, and finally the necessity of social services. (1963: #9, #11)

To be in accordance with the dignity of the human person, therefore, necessary health care must be as available as is reasonably possible in a manner that does not discriminate on the basis of wealth, social status, age, sex, or race. Health care providers must treat individuals as being capable, under the proper circumstances, of making free and responsible choices, as well as having the human, social, and religious obligation to do so. Health care that denies either explicitly or implicitly the freedom or intelligence of the human person would not be in accordance with Catholic social teaching; likewise, health care that treats human freedom as an absolute, or that pretends that society does not have a legitimate interest in the choices that individuals make, would also be out of kilter with Catholic social teaching. Health care must deal with the whole person--physical, emotional, rational,

---

for thoughtful appraisal of complex problems and acknowledges that some problems can only be addressed effectively at the national level. This principle recognizes the importance of interpersonal relationships and the need for individuals to be engaged in efforts to improve their social condition.

responsible, capable of loving, social--and at the same time be realistically in touch with both human limitations and human potentials.

Authentic Human Development

Catholic social teaching has stressed that authentic human development includes both a material and a spiritual dimension. Hope in eternal life does not diminish but rather increases our concern for justice in this life. One should neither neglect the material in favor of the purely spiritual, nor neglect the spiritual in favor of exclusively material concerns. This emphasis in Catholic social teaching can be linked with contemporary holistic approaches to health care that treat the whole person: physical, mental, and spiritual.

In *Sollicitudo Rei Socialis* (1987), John Paul II draws upon the opening chapters of Genesis to demonstrate that human beings are composed of both body and soul:

> . . .in trying to achieve true development we must never lose sight of that *dimension* which is the *specific nature* of human beings, who have been created by God in God's image and likeness (cf. Gen 1:26). It is a bodily and a spiritual nature, symbolized in the second creation account by the two elements: the *earth*, from which God forms the man's body, and the *breath of life*, which God breathes into the man's nostrils. (cf: Gen 2:7) (John Paul II, Pope, 1987: #29)

Human beings are thus creatures who have a certain affinity with other creatures, but at the same time are called in a special way to be subject to the will of God.

Human development thereby has a moral dimension. On the one hand, a great stress must be placed upon the freedom and responsibility of the individual person. Approaches to social problems that simply treat individuals as helpless victims without eliciting personal commitment on their part would not be in harmony with Catholic social teaching.

On the other hand, John Paul II stresses just as strongly that commitment to human development "is not just an *individual* duty, still less an *individualistic* one, as if it were possible to achieve this development through the isolated efforts of individuals" (1987: #32). Human freedom must therefore be linked with the reality of human interconnectedness and recognize the duty "*of all towards all*" (1987: #32). Thus approaches to social problems that place unrealistic expectations upon individuals without accounting for the complexities of social, economic, and political factors would be no more in harmony with Catholic social teaching than approaches that ignore individual responsibility.

John Paul II thus calls both for an appreciation of individual responsibility and for a recognition of human interconnectedness: "In order to be genuine, human development must be achieved within the framework of *solidarity* and *freedom*, without ever sacrificing either of them under whatever pretext" (1987: #33). Solidarity involves the firm commitment of all to the common good, "because we are *all* really responsible for *all*" (John Paul II, Pope, 1987: #38). John Paul II goes so far as to link solidarity with charity, the foremost of Christian virtues:

> *Solidarity* is undoubtedly a *Christian_virtue*. In what has been said so far it has been possible to identify many points of contact between solidarity and *charity*, which is the distinguishing mark of Christ's disciples. (cf. John 13:35) (1987: #40)

The implications of John Paul II's reflections for adolescent health care are many. Practical circumstances in our pluralistic society call for approaches that minimize the use of explicitly religious terminology; however, to be in harmony with Catholic social teaching, health care must address the needs of the entire person, physical, mental, and spiritual, in a holistic manner. Attention must be given to value development and character formation. Those elements of human life traditionally addressed by the world's major religions, such as basic life orientation, values, ultimate meaning, *raison d'etre*, basic morals, respect for social conventions, and personal discipline, cannot be ignored in the face of social pathologies that place at risk the health of millions of individuals and that are eroding the common good. At the same time, any focus on the individual must be balanced by a vision that considers the larger community and social context. Catholic social teaching thus calls for pressing problems to be addressed with creative solutions that combine individual responsibility with community and social support.

The Common Good

While striving to ensure the dignity of all persons, Catholic teaching points out that human dignity is attained in association with others; it is realized in community with others (National Conference of Catholic Bishops, 1984: #23). Thus the dignity of the human person is placed in a social context and involves an obligation on the part of each person to support others in society. The Catholic tradition affirms that:

> each person is sustained and nourished by his or her integration with, and

dependence on, the whole community. Our thoroughly social nature entails an obligation to serve the common good . (Catholic Health Association, 1992: 3)

The "common good" in Catholic thought refers neither to the needs and wants of the majority nor those of a vocal minority, but rather to the greatest good for the greatest number (National Conference of Catholic Bishops, 1986: #80).

This concept of the common good poses an especially great challenge for those in American society. Historically, Americans have supported a stronger sense of individualism than of communitarian spirit. This individualism is a common theme throughout American culture and is well illustrated by such admonitions as "pull yourself up by the bootstraps" and "every man for himself" (Bellah, Madsen, Sullivan, Swidler, & Tipton, 1985). Catholic teaching presents a contrasting world-view which places a strong emphasis on the community.

A Catholic approach will emphasize that as members of society, individuals have rights and responsibilities toward themselves and toward others. These rights include the right to life and to all that makes life human. Put negatively, "any denial of these rights [to food, clothing, shelter, medical care] harms persons and wounds the human community" (National Conference of Catholic Bishops, 1986: #80). Furthermore, individuals also have the responsibility to take care of themselves, their families, and others. To respect the rights and needs of others is, in essence, to work for the common good.

While an understanding of the need for service toward the common good is not new, it has often been overlooked in the United States. Nevertheless, the value of common good probably presents the most succinct moral standard by which the actions of organizations and individuals in society can be measured. This principle suggests that society and its members have an obligation to pursue developing a full range of organizations which better serve the common good.

This obligation calls for a complex and multifaceted response that would entail a collaboration and commitment from all sectors of society. In the case of health care, it suggests that it is the responsibility of the health care providers, patients, and their families, the insurance industry, schools, and government to discover ways to better utilize resources so that better health care services will be available to more members of society.

The Centrality of the Family

From the early Church, and continuing through contemporary Catholic social teaching, the integrity and intrinsic value of the family has been a central principle. Catholic tradition presents the family unit as "incarnational"--a primary vehicle for God's activity in the world. It is the function of the family to nourish, sustain, and provide its members with an understanding of their relationship with God and of their role in society. The family is thus sometimes called the "church of the home" or the "domestic church"; it is the primary site of faith formation.

A contemporary approach to family has been articulated in *Gaudium et Spes* (Vatican Council II, 1965) and in *Familiaris Consortio* (John Paul II, Pope, 1981). The family is here presented as the most basic foundation of the Church, of society, and of all human communities. John Paul II sums this up in his address to the Confederacy of Family Advisory Bureaus of Christian Inspiration: "The future of the world and of the church passes through the family" (John Paul II, Pope 1980). In *Familaris Consortio*, he elaborates on this point:

> The family is the first and fundamental school of social living: As a community of love, it finds in self-giving the law that guides it and makes it grow. The self-giving that inspires the love of husband and wife for each other is the model and norm for the self-giving that must be practiced in the relationships between brothers and sisters and the different generations living together in the family. And the communion and sharing that are part of everyday life in the home at times of joy and at times of difficulty are the most concrete and effective pedagogy for the active, responsible and fruitful inclusion of the children in the wider horizon of society. (1981: #37)

Although the Church upholds the family as vital, it is also cognizant of the changing social context in which the family exists. As we have moved from an agricultural society to a post-industrial or neo-capitalist society, the rights and responsibilities of the family in society have changed. Society has become increasingly complex; families have become increasingly interdependent on other institutions, organizations, and government. Families are no longer able to meet all of the needs of their members. For example, families are now dependent on other organizations to meet many of the health care needs of their members. As families become increasingly interdependent on these other social organizations, it is essential to remember that "the family exists prior to the State or any other community and possesses rights which are inalienable" (The Vatican, 1983: Preamble: 1). In considering the role of the family in society, John Paul II stated, "No plan of organized pastoral work at any level must fail to take into consideration the pastoral area of the family" (1981: 68).

Ethical approaches to human sexual behavior in harmony with Catholic social teaching take on their full meaning only against the backdrop of an affirmation of the importance, and even sacredness, of marriage and the family. Proscriptions against premarital and other forms of nonmarital sexual behaviors simply do not make sense within an individualistic consumer mentality that looks to cost-benefits and demands, "show me what's wrong with it." Fostering appropriate values among adolescents regarding sexuality goes hand in hand with fostering appropriate values regarding marriage and the family.

Preparation for family life can no longer be simply the job of the family, as it had been in traditional societies. John Paul II argues that "the changes that have taken place within almost all modern societies demand that not only the family but also society and the church should be involved in the effort of properly preparing young people for their future responsibilities" (1981: #66). In accordance with this understanding, he places a good deal of emphasis on marriage preparation.[40]

The family and society are not adversaries; rather, they have complementary functions with the common goals of supporting their members and fostering the common good. Families and institutions have resources and responsibilities that reflect their interdependence. The Catholic tradition, then, acknowledges the central and unique role of the family in society as well as its interdependence with a full range of other social institutions. It is the responsibility of those shaping these other social organizations and institutions to recognize the primacy of the family and to develop forms responsive to the needs of the families of its members. When the primacy of the family is considered by health care providers, for example, the patient is not viewed in isolation but rather as a member of a family. In the case of adolescents, treatment will often involve the parents, spouse, or children of the patient. Such family involvement can be expected to be especially helpful whenever the illness or problem is tied to lifestyle choices, cultural habits, or a particular worldview.

---

[40] John Paul II identifies three stages of marriage preparation: remote, proximate, and immediate. Remote preparation begins in early childhood and includes esteem for human values, a basic respect for marriage, and a proper attitude toward those of the opposite sex. The proximate preparation "will present marriage as an interpersonal relationship of a man and a woman that has to be continually developed, and it will encourage those concerned to study the nature of conjugal sexuality and responsible parenthood, with the essential medical and biological knowledge connected with it" (1981: #66). The immediate preparation will be more intense and help give marriage more meaning and purpose.

Preferential Option for the Poor

A concern for social justice, including just treatment of the powerless, can be traced back to a number of passages in the Old Testament (Exodus 22: 21-27, Deuteronomy 15: 1-11, Job 29: 11-17, Ezekiel 22: 21-27). In the New Testament, Jesus is consistently portrayed as one who reached out to the socially marginalized and disenfranchised. This theme was expressed by Leo XIII in *Rerum Novarum:*

> . . .the favor of God himself seems to incline more toward the unfortunate as a class; for Jesus Christ calls the poor blessed, and he invites most lovingly all who are in labor or sorrow to come to him, embracing with special love the lowly and those harassed by injustice. (1939: #37)

This "option for the poor" has become a rallying cry not only for theologians and bishops of Latin America, but also for John Paul II, who, in an address to the Brazilian bishops, described it as a

> call to have a special openness with the small and weak, those that suffer and weep, those that are humiliated and left on the margins of society, so as to help them with their dignity as human persons and as children of God. (*Origins*, 1980: 135)

The preferential option for the poor is basically a matter of justice in social context. It includes but is more than simply "taking care of" the poor. In their pastoral letter on the economy, the U.S. bishops said that:

> . . .we should seek solutions that enable the poor to help themselves through such means as employment. Paternalistic programs which do too much for the poor and too little with the poor are to be avoided. (National Conference of Catholic Bishops, 1986: #188)

They argue that the appropriate goal "is to enable *all* persons to share in and contribute to the common good" (National Conference of Catholic Bishops, 1986: #87); this goal entails the obligation to help the poor to become active and productive (National Conference of Catholic Bishops, 1986: #86).

The bishops draw from the example of Jesus and argue that the preferential option for the poor involves the following challenges:

> It imposes a prophetic mandate to speak for those who have no one to speak for them, to be a defender of the defenseless who, in biblical terms, are the poor. It also demands a compassionate vision which enables the Church to see things from the side of the poor and powerless, to assess

lifestyle, policy, and social institutions and policies in terms of their impact on the poor. It summons the Church also to be an instrument in assisting people to experience the liberating power of God in their own lives so that they may respond to the gospel in freedom and in dignity. Finally, and most radically, it calls for an emptying of self, both individually and corporatively, that allows the Church to experience the power of God in the midst of poverty and powerlessness. (National Conference of Catholic Bishops, 1986: #52)

Recent studies have confirmed that the fastest growing segment of the poor in the United States is young people (Children's Defense Fund, 1991). A neglect of the poor and the marginalized constitutes a threat to their human dignity: "the society that neglects them places their conscience at risk" (Catholic Health Association, 1991: 17). This principle of Church teaching calls for individuals and social organizations to make a commitment to "to speak for the voiceless," and "to defend the defenseless" (National Conference of Catholic Bishops, 1986: #16).

One of the crucial difficulties of poverty in the United States is the inadequacy of health care for poor persons. A relatively high percentage of poor children are not immunized against preventable childhood diseases (Children's Defense Fund, 1991). Many of those in poverty are unable to afford adequate health care or live in areas where it is largely inaccessible. Yet this Catholic social teaching would suggest that it is precisely the treatment of these individuals--those most vulnerable in society--by which the health care service system should be evaluated.

Subsidiarity

It could be argued that the Catholic social principle of subsidiarity can be traced in the workings of God and in the response of human beings throughout scripture and tradition. However, this principle has its modern birth in the 1891 encyclical *Rerum Novarum* (Leo XIII, Pope, 1939) and the actual term was first used in 1931 in *Quadragesimo Anno* (Pius XI, Pope, 1931). This modern notion of subsidiarity began as an endorsement of the basic idea underlying labor unions: that people can organize and network in a face-to-face manner to support each other and to work collectively to create better social conditions.

The most basic meaning of the term "subsidiarity" is that social problems should be addressed on the lowest level of organization possible.[41]

---

[41] The term "subsidarity" is also used by secular social ethicists when explaining the appropriate role of the state in society. According to Sheeran, "(s)tates

Local problems should be tackled at the local level. Regional, state, and national programs should support rather than replace local efforts. It is not enough to throw money at problems in an impersonal manner and then turn away. People need to be empowered as individuals to participate in organized endeavors to improve social conditions.

This is not to devalue regional or state or national or international programs and support. Surely problems exist that call for solutions on such levels of organization. Subsidiarity is rather a call to place a primary emphasis on people networking together on local levels to make a difference in the quality of life available to those most in need. Local efforts tend to be more personal and more in touch with the specific needs of individuals and groups than are programs run on larger levels. An emphasis on empowering people to participate in local solutions helps larger programs be faithful to the teaching of *Gaudium et Spes* that "the subject and goal of all social institutions is and must be the human person" (Vatican Council II, 1965: #25).

In terms of adolescent health care, this principle calls for a strategy of service delivery that empowers adolescents and their families to maintain or obtain health and well-being that is responsive to the specifics of their life-conditions. It calls for the support or development of health care institutions that emphasize the importance of local-level involvement in their structure, control, and organization. A health-care system run from the national or state level with little local autonomy is unlikely to grasp the vast variety of adolescent health problems. A health-care system controlled by the medical professionals with little input from the patients and their families undermines any efforts at empowerment; people who have no control over their health or no say in the treatment they receive are unlikely to develop health-conscious behaviors.

Consistent Ethic of Life

Any approach to health care that is in harmony with Catholic social teaching will uphold an ethic that respects life. The sacredness and the dignity of each human life is to be championed. A foundation for such an approach was articulated forcefully in *Gaudium et Spes*:

---

exist to help people do what they are unable to do for themselves. This is the principle of subsidiarity--that the state should never do for its citizens what the citizens can do for themselves. In practice, it means that the state should help its citizens only when they need help. It should supplement, not supplant. In this capacity, the state is acting for the common good" (1993: 137).

. . .whatever is opposed to life itself, such as any type of murder, genocide, abortion, euthanasia or willful self-destruction, whatever violates the integrity of the human person, such as mutilation, torments inflicted on body or mind, attempts to coerce the will itself; whatever insults human dignity, such as subhuman living conditions, arbitrary imprisonment, deportation, slavery, prostitution, the selling of women and children; as well as disgraceful working conditions, where men are treated as mere tools for profit, rather than as free and responsible persons; all these things and others of their like are infamies indeed. (Vatican Council II, 1965: #27)

Over the past decade, Cardinal Bernardin of Chicago has worked toward the development of a consistent ethic of life. The consistent life ethic "cuts across the issues of genetics, abortion, capital punishment, modern warfare and the care of the terminally ill" (Bernardin, 1983: 493). It is based on the premise that "success on any one of these issues requires a concern for the broader attitudes in society about respect for human life" (Bernardin, 1983: 493). The various life issues all fit together in such a way that if people examine deeply enough the rationale underlying a life-stance that they take on any one issue, they will be forced to consider whether their positions on other issues build consistently upon the same principles. Thus opposition to capital punishment, if consistent, implies opposition to abortion; opposition to abortion implies a commitment to the improvement of social conditions. All rests upon the sacred dignity of the human person.

Approaches to health care in harmony with Catholic social teaching will establish ethical policies that reflect a consistent life ethic. This will involve not only a witness against individual deeds that directly violate the consistent life ethic, but also a strong commitment to take action in alleviating social circumstances that diminish human dignity. For example, it is not enough to be opposed to abortion; one truly opposed to abortion will also be concerned about social and economic problems that can make abortion appear to be an attractive solution to an otherwise hopeless person. Cardinal Bernardin has clarified that any one individual might choose to concentrate solely on one issue for the sake of effectiveness; such a person, however, should be aware of the deep interconnectedness of the various ills that violate human dignity (Bernardin, 1984: 708-09).

Cardinal Bernardin has recently applied the consistent ethic of life to the current health care debate. Bernardin distinguishes between, on the one hand, universal <u>access</u> to health care coverage and, on the other hand, actual universal health care coverage along with the practical means of obtaining it. The former, he argues, is not enough. Only the latter is in harmony with a consistent life ethic that acknowledges health care as "an essential safeguard of human dignity" (Bernardin, 1994: 7). Bernardin argues further that the allocation of scarce health care resources must:

be oriented to the common good, apply to all, result from an open and participatory process, give priority to disadvantaged persons, be free of wrongful discrimination, and be monitored in its social and economic effects. (1994: 9)

Finally, Bernardin argues that any morally acceptable plan must reject any mandate to include abortion.

An approach to health care in harmony with Catholic teaching will oppose both abortion and euthanasia. At the same time it will address social conditions, such as sub-human standards of living, that violate the dignity of the human person.

A Public Voice

Cardinal Bernardin has argued that the consistent ethic of life represents an appropriate posture for Catholic teaching in public forums. For Catholics it is religiously based, for it grows out of faith and tradition. At the same time, however, it can be argued for persuasively on the basis of respect for life without using explicitly religious arguments. It has an inherent appeal to many in the public sphere from various backgrounds of belief and outlook. Cardinal Bernardin urges that Catholics retain their religious grounding as they seek ways of expressing themselves that move the public conversation forward while being sensitive to pluralism.

Bernardin proposes a vision of human rights that both affirms and challenges certain elements of American culture. He outlines a view that places individual rights and duties within a communal framework:

> These convictions find their origin in a vision of the human person as someone who is grounded in community, and in an understanding of society and government as being largely responsible for the realization of the common good. As Catholics we share this vision with many others. It is consistent with fundamental American values, though grounded differently. For example, our Declaration of Independence and our Constitution reflect a profound insight that has guided the development of our nation; namely, that there are certain fundamental human rights that exist before the creation of any social contract (such as the constitution of a sovereign nation), and that these must be protected by society and government. There is an objective order to which we are held accountable and to which we, in turn, hold others accountable in our many relationships and activities. The Catholic tradition also affirms such rights but sees them emerging from the organic relationship between the individual and the community. (Bernardin, 1994: 5)

Bernardin's vision reflects the position on the relationship between the individual and community found in Leo XIII's *Rerum Novarum* (1939) as well in subsequent Catholic social teaching. Though not politically partisan, it also has much in common with the "democratic communitarian"[42] outlook articulated by sociologist Robert Bellah (1994), who draws upon the work of Jonathan Boswell (1990). These views also coincide with the "moderate communitarianism" advocated by Kenneth Himes and Michael Himes from a more theological perspective (1993).

These communitarian thinkers interact creatively with the philosophically liberal political stances of our times, whether the conservative libertarianism of a Robert Nozick or the modern liberalism of a John Rawls, that emphasize the rights of individuals in a way that is prior to any social contract. Bellah and the Himes brothers argue that not just individuals but also certain types of communities, such as families and neighborhoods, exist prior to more complicated levels of social organization and have their own rights and responsibilities. In a communitarian vision, the individual, while extremely important, is understood not as an isolated atom but relationally, as being formed within and remaining in relation to various types of communities.

A moderate communitarian vision respects individual rights but does not place them categorically above the rights of communities and the common good. In contrast to philosophically liberal approaches that label moral issues as private and personal and push them out of public discussion, a communitarian vision demands that on crucial issues a moral consensus be sought in the public sphere. A community that achieves a degree of consensus can regulate its standards both legally and culturally; that is, through both legislation and the shaping of attitudes and values in the public sphere. In this vision, abortion is not simply an individual's private right. Pornography in neighborhood stores is not just another convenience for consumers. The growing gap between the rich and the poor cannot simply be written off as an unfortunate consequence of the best of all possible economic systems.

An example of an issue that cries out for public consensus in the face of social deterioration can be found in the work of Karla Brent Hackstaff (1994; as discussed in Bellah, 1994). Hackstaff contrasts characteristics of a "marriage culture" with those of a "divorce culture." In the former, marriage is a given, is expected to be permanent, and divorce is a last resort.

---

[42]   Communitarianism is a philosophy which emphasizes the need for an active, value-based, citizen participation in the large structures of the economy and the state. It highlights the argument that "the common good of the community should take precedence over self-interested, autonomous individuals" (Sjoberg, Williams, Gill, & Himmel, 1995: 248).

In the latter, marriage is an option, its length is contingent, and divorce is often seen as a liberating gateway to a more fulfilling life. Hackstaff finds in her study that at this time the divorce culture represents a significant challenge to, but has not yet replaced, the marriage culture. She concludes that the emerging divorce culture is caused less by new roles for women in society than by the failure of men to meet women's rising expectations for male participation in marriage and family.

A relevant question raised by Hackstaff's work is whether cultural trends such as the rise of a divorce culture can be identified, analyzed, and opted against by various groups, associations, and communities within our society. Can a public consensus be reached that the marriage culture is to be preferred over the divorce culture? Could there exist, for example, health care alternatives that are conscious of such cultural problems and that self-consciously help to work toward their resolution?

Many cautions are necessary in this approach. Bellah clarifies that in the democratic communitarian view, individual rights remain very important. He is willing, for example, to acknowledge the first premise of the divorce culture, that marriage is today an option, not a given (Bellah, 1994: 16). Also, he insists that he is not advocating a romantic return to a past when roles were rigidly defined and repressively enforced. But he argues that certain elements of our culture that used to be taken for granted, even marriage itself, will not survive unless people take conscious and positive responsibility for promoting and safeguarding them. Such support will come through legislation, through economic policy, and through a reappropriation of traditional virtues into contemporary communities.

Catholic social teaching lends support to the quest for public consensus on moral issues. In relation to adolescent health care, this would involve developing strategies for reinforcing positive elements of the adolescent sub-culture as well as challenging negative elements. No plan for adolescent health care, no matter how comprehensive, can be expected to do this alone. It must work in conjunction with a wide network of communities. But if some degree of public consensus on a range of key issues could be forged, then those who work in adolescent health care could be significant contributors in shaping the culture of teens.

Hope

Hope is a major theme that runs throughout Catholic teaching. Classically, hope has been understood as the mean between the extremes of presumption and despair. In contemporary Catholic social teaching hope is the rejection, on the one hand, of the attitude of those who allow themselves to be overwhelmed by the enormity of the problems that we face as a society; on the other hand, hope is the rejection of the attitude of those who think that the reality that we have now really isn't so bad, that current conditions are acceptable, that we are as close to the coming of the kingdom as we need to be for now. *Gaudium et Spes* calls Christians to embrace hope in anticipation of the coming of God's kingdom:

> . . .while we are warned that it profits one nothing if one gains the whole world and loses oneself, the expectation of a new earth must not weaken but rather stimulate our concern for cultivating this one. For here grows the body of a new human family, a body which even now is able to give some kind of foreshadowing of the new age. (Vatican Council II, 1965: #39)

Hope, therefore, is the attitude with which this report now returns to a consideration of the pragmatic difficulties faced by those wishing to improve adolescent health and of the strategies we will develop, hopefully, to resolve those difficulties and meet the challenge of adolescent health.

CHAPTER 4

THE DELIVERY OF ADOLESCENT HEALTH CARE

The health care needs of adolescents include all of the biomedical conditions, developmental conditions tied to their maturation, and the social morbidities characteristic of a teenager's life in America. The medical needs of adolescents are diverse and complex; often they appear in clusters and they are almost always closely tied to the social situations of the young people. In many cases, these medical needs are not being met.

The American College of Physicians has concluded that adolescents, as a group, are medically under-served for a number of reasons (Snyder, 1989). The reasons they cite include an insufficient number of providers trained in adolescent health care, a lack of emphasis on health-promoting education, and limited financial reimbursement for adolescent care. Others assert that the main barrier to health care is purely financial; many adolescents do not have access to private health insurance or to services funded by the government. Some physicians point out that the time needed to manage adolescent problems exceeds that needed for most other populations, thus exacerbating the problem of limited financial reimbursement (Blum, 1987b). The delivery of health-care services to adolescents is further complicated by the very structure of the social and medical services needed. The diversity of health problems experienced by adolescents requires an extensive system of prevention and treatment that takes into account the interrelationships among various health problems. The current health care system consists of a patchwork of programs that vary greatly in their ability to provide appropriate and accessible care. Adolescents are also under-served due to the inability (or unwillingness) of health-care providers to view adolescents' health care as a family-centered activity. Very often the family systems which impinge upon or support adolescents' health-related behaviors are not factored into the analysis of the problem.   The lack of family-oriented services often results in counterproductive or otherwise ineffective treatments for adolescents' health problems.

Efficient and adequate delivery of health services to adolescents is also hampered by a series of physical, communication, and perception difficulties. For example, some minority youth find the health care system particularly unsupportive; cultural assumptions on the part of the practitioners may be direct affronts to those of minority teens and their families. Adolescents whose primary physician is a pediatrician may have difficulty with the physical setting of the doctor's office. Some health providers may have most of their office hours during the normal school day while others may be difficult to reach by public transportation. Some adolescents may be afraid to access available services because they believe that others will view them as "crazy," "a drug addict," or "a slut".

The theological considerations of the preceding chapter suggest that, despite the complexity, we need to recognize the barriers to good health care for adolescents and to attempt to remove them. Doing so requires looking for solutions that both respect the individual dignity of adolescents and recognize their place as members of a community; most specifically, as members of families. Theology can provide only guidelines, rather than concrete solutions to medical problems, but its guidance is crucial in choosing among a variety of alternatives.

USE OF HEALTH CARE SERVICES BY ADOLESCENTS

According to one national study, 72% of 10- to 18-year-olds had at least one visit with a physician during 1986 (Gans, McManus, & Newacheck, 1991). Another study indicates that, on average, each adolescent in this country visited a physician 1.6 times during 1985 (U.S. Congress, Office of Technology Assessment, 1991c: 9); yet another suggests an average of 3 visits per year for each teen (Gans, McManus, & Newacheck, 1991). These visits include screenings for participation in organized sports and concern all types of ailments from acne to gunshot wounds. They include the treatment of acute conditions, chronic problems, mental health difficulties, and preventative care.

Conversely, however, not all adolescents receive the treatment they need nor the yearly preventative physician contact recommended by the

American Medical Association.[43] Many do not have an opportunity to see a physician for long periods of time. Results from the National Health Interview Survey in 1988 indicate that nearly one quarter of U.S. 12- to 17-year-olds had not seen a physician in over one year.[44] Another study indicates that in 1986, some four million adolescents (14%) had no contact with a physician for more than two years (Gans, McManus, & Newacheck, 1991).

FIGURE 4.1:   Visits to Private Office-Based Physicians by U.S. Adolescents Ages 10 to 18, by Duration of Visit, 1985 (estimated N = 50,218,000)

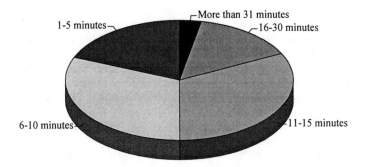

SOURCE: U.S. Department of Health and Human Services, Public Health Service, Centers for Disease Control, National Center for Health Statistics, unpublished data from the 1985 National Ambulatory Medical Care Survey, Hyattsville MD, 1989. Cited in U.S. Congress, Office of Technology Assessment, *Adolescent health-Volume III: Crosscutting issues in the delivery of health and related services,* 1991c: 12.

---

[43] For more information concerning the preventative services recommended by the American Medical Association, see Figure 15 of this document or American Medical Association, 1992.

[44] Similar results are cited by Cromer from four other surveys of teens in the United States and Canada (1992).

Despite the seriousness of many of the presenting ailments, many of the visits teens do have with private physicians are relatively short. While many diagnoses can accurately be made very quickly, a five-minute appointment does not allow for much anticipatory guidance (preventative care) especially for many of the complex conditions facing adolescents such as their participation in early sexual activity, alcohol abuse, or excessive risk-taking. As can be seen in Figure 4.1, fewer than a quarter of all visits are more than 15 minutes in duration (U.S. Congress, Office of Technology Assessment, 1991c). Time constraints undoubtedly serve to limit the viability of physicians' prevention and counseling efforts as well as their ability to identify accurately the underlying causes of adolescents' health problems.

Variations by Income

Long gaps between visits to a physician and the likelihood of hospitalization are tied to the economic condition of the adolescent's family. Gans, McManus, & Newacheck point out that poor adolescents are 1.2 times more likely than nonpoor teens to have 2 or more years elapse between physician visits (1991: 6). As Cromer points out, given the increased prevalence of many of the serious social morbidities:

> among families living in poverty, it would seem particularly important that the adolescents in such families present for medical and behavioral assessment. Data from national surveys, however, suggest a positive relationship between low socioeconomic status and poor health care utilization. Additionally, brief physical examinations for the purpose of determining eligibility for sports participation (usually performed *en masse* in a gymnasium without attention to other medical or psychosocial issues) often supplant the annual checkup; in one survey, the sports evaluation represented the only contact with the medical system for over 75% of participating students. (1992: 30)

Perhaps because of the dearth of preventative and primary care among the poor, young people from poor families are more likely than nonpoor teens to have been hospitalized during the course of the year.[45] The National Health Interview Survey, for instance, indicates that children and

---

[45] In general, adolescents have hospitalization rates well below those of most other age groups. Approximately 5% of female and 3% of male 12- to 17-year-olds were hospitalized in 1986 (Adams & Hardy, 1989; Gans, McManus, & Newacheck, 1991).

adolescents under 18 with household incomes of under $10,000 annually were hospitalized at a rate of 5.8 per 100 individuals.[46] For young people with family incomes of $35,000 or more, the comparable rate was 2.8 (U.S. Congress, Office of Technology Assessment, 1991c: III-12). These data also indicate that economically disadvantaged young people on average also spend more days in the hospital for each stay. The average length of stay for those in families with incomes under $10,000 is 6.9 days while for those in families earning more than $35,000 annually the average hospital stay is 4.6 days. Nonpoor adolescents are more than 1.5 times more likely than those who are poor to have received dental care within the year.

Variations Among Minorities

Despite having worse health status than white teens, health care services are not accessed as readily nor as often by nonwhites and Latinos (Andersen, Giachello, & Aday, 1986; Gans, McManus, & Newacheck, 1991; Lieu, Newacheck, & McManus, 1993; Mendoza, Martorell, & Castillo, 1989; U.S. Congress, Office of Technology Assessment, 1991c; U.S. Department of Health and Human Services, 1990). Some of this variation is tied to differences in income; some to disparities in insurance status. Lieu, Newacheck, and McManus, however, in their recent analysis of the National Health Interview Survey, conclude that persistent racial differences in access to health care remain even after controlling for health insurance, family income, health status, and other factors (1993: 960).

These persistent and pervasive inequities in health care delivery mirror, of course, inequities in society as a whole. Their entrenched nature and diffuse effect should not discourage those committed to the dignity of the individual and to the common good from continuing to search for creative ways to remedy the situation.

BARRIERS TO THE DELIVERY AND USE OF HEALTH SERVICES

Several factors prevent adolescents from accessing effective health care and from perceiving services as approachable or appropriate to their needs. Six will be addressed in this document. Most fundamental is the limited

---

[46] The National Health Interview Survey included a child health supplement for 7465 10- to 17-year-olds (Lieu, Newacheck, McManus, 1993).

availability of health care providers who understand the unique needs of adolescents; as we have seen, the health needs of teenagers are somewhat different from those of adults and of younger children. Secondly, the fragmented nature of the health care system is a barrier to effective service delivery to adolescents. A third barrier entails the individual orientation of the health care system; it is not family-centered. Fourth, the health care services offered to adolescents often do not effectively take into consideration the needs, tastes, skills, and abilities of their particular patients. Another important barrier to the efficient delivery and use of health care services is the cultural differences that make diagnosis and treatment of some adolescents substantially different than others. The sixth barrier to the delivery of health care to youth is the inability of many to pay for services.

Limited Availability of Trained Health Providers and Services

No one group of primary care physicians is clearly defined as appropriate to provide care for adolescents. Adolescents are most likely to visit family practice physicians or pediatricians (DuRant, 1991; U.S. Congress, Office of Technology Assessment, 1991b). According to Office of Technology Assessment figures (1991a, 1991b), 1,400-2,000 primary care physicians specialize in adolescent care and 1,500 psychologists, 1,500 psychiatrists, and 370 obstetrician-gynecologists express a specific interest in adolescents. Large percentages of primary care physicians perceive themselves as insufficiently trained to diagnose and treat adolescent health problems (Blum, 1987a; U.S. Congress, Office of Technology Assessment, 1991a, 1991b).

In one study, physicians who often treat adolescents (internists, pediatricians, and family practitioners) rated their competency in a number of areas of adolescent health care. They found themselves to be especially ill-prepared to treat social morbidities such as drug or alcohol abuse and eating disorders (Blum, 1987b). Nearly half of the physicians surveyed for this study report deficiencies in their training in areas of social concerns or mental health such as depression, suicide, and family conflicts (Blum, 1987b). In addition, relatively few physicians indicate an interest in obtaining additional training to work with adolescents (Blum, 1987b; U.S. Congress, Office of Technology Assessment, 1991b). As Figure 4.2 illustrates, nurses, social workers, and psychologists also consider themselves untrained in important areas of adolescent health (U.S. Congress, Office of Technology Assessment, 1991b; U.S. Congress, Office of Technology Assessment, 1991c).

FIGURE 4.2:   Percent of Surveyed Health Professionals Who Perceive Themselves to be Insufficiently Trained to Manage Adolescents' Health Issues, by Respondents' Professional Discipline (N = 1660)

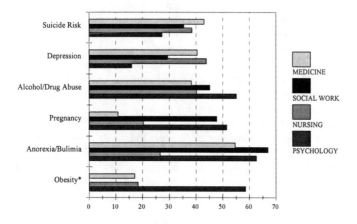

* Social workers were not asked this question.

SOURCE: Adapted by permission of Elsevier Science Inc. from "Knowledge and attitudes of health professionals toward adolescent health care" by Blum & Bearinger, *Journal of Adolescent Health Care*, Vol. 11, No. 4, pp. 290. Copyright 1990 by the Society for Adolescent Medicine.

A number of studies indicate that those physicians who do regularly treat adolescents are often not able to identify emotional problems, behavior problems, or substance use and abuse problems in their patients (U.S. Congress, Office of Technology Assessment, 1991c). Some research suggests that primary care physicians may not identify a high proportion of existent emotional and behavioral problems not only because of patient bias against the diagnosis and limited physician preparation, but because the time spent with the patients is often insufficient to adequately assess the situation (Costello, Edlebrock, Costello, Dulcan, Burns & Brent, 1988; Chang, Warner, Weissman, 1988; Chang & Astrachan, 1988; Kamerow, Pincus, & MacDonald, 1986).

Fragmentation of Services

The United States has a complex public and private system of health care services designed to assist individuals and families. These services are provided by a wide range of organizations including government agencies, private nonprofit organizations, schools, employers, community-based organizations, religious organizations, and informal networks of friends and relatives. Many of these organizations provide one or more narrowly-defined health care services to a narrowly-defined group of clients. Public health departments, for example, often run separate facilities for specific public health needs such as tuberculosis, sexually transmitted diseases, immunizations, sickle cell disease, and prenatal programs. Adolescent clients may warrant simultaneous service at a number of such facilities but be unable to manage such a complex system.

Despite the fragmentation and lack of coordination inherent in such an approach, these organizations often meet the needs of many adults who have a specific illness or difficulty. In the case of adolescent health care, however, the lack of integrated policy, programs, and service delivery results in inefficient and inadequate service delivery to the teens, a compounding of problems within their families, and increased costs of services that must address problems after they have worsened.

With the exception of a few preventative programs, current health and social service delivery systems often do not deal effectively with adolescents. The service-delivery systems are especially ill-equipped to deal with those who are experiencing multiple, interrelated difficulties. In such a situation, a focused program may alleviate one specific problem but be unable to assess and treat the broader syndrome of problems affecting a given family or individual. Some problems presented to a given health care provider may be symptoms of other problems; for example, those who have frequent urinary or gynecological problems may be sexually active or subject to sexual abuse. Children having school problems may be living in a family beset with violence, substance abuse or other problems; those who consistently do not complete their school work may be clinically depressed or employed so many hours each week that they suffer from exhaustion.

Some adolescents fare better than others in overcoming the fragmentation of health care services; some are subject to special difficulties. Young people who are poor, those with multiple health problems, those with dysfunctional family situations, and those with physical or mental handicaps find negotiating the health care system to be especially problematic. Certainly those adolescents who have access to sufficient financial resources generally manage to piece together some health care services. For those adolescents with fewer resources, however, the task is much more formidable. In addition, adolescents whose families experience multiple, severe problems also are less likely than others to have the skills and resources necessary to identify and gain access to the multiple services needed to address their complex problems.   Without integration, whole groups of young people are not likely to receive appropriate medical care. Consider, for instance, the care of handicapped youth. As Haggerty, Roghmann, and Pless (1993) point out, in many areas of the country severely handicapped adolescents are treated by specialists rather than by a primary care team:

> Primary care physicians (pediatricians or family physicians) often are unwilling to provide even general care for the child with severe handicaps (e.g., patients with spina bifida), yet sub-specialty clinics, usually well set up for technical care, do not ordinarily provide preventative services, nor do they take responsibility for 24-hour-a-day comprehensive care. (322)

Similarly, those clearly needing mental health care generally cannot receive integrated services. Despite the influence of social-psychological ailments on the biomedical condition of adolescents, the treatment of physical and mental difficulties often is poorly coordinated. Effective integration would involve communication and collaboration across subspecialties, institutions, and organizations.

These families and the adolescents in them need comprehensive, coordinated, and intensive assistance that is not available in an uncoordinated service delivery system made up of autonomous, narrowly defined programs. They need integrated and sustained interventions delivered by professionals who recognize and are able to respond to a family's multiple problems and needs (National Commission on Children, 1991). They need programs that focus on the needs of clients rather than programs developed in response to policy that focuses on one area of concern and fails to address the interrelationship of that particular concern and other problem areas also experienced by the target group of the policy. Once again, a theology committed to the dignity of the individual can provide a rationale and inspiration for keeping the focus of such programs where they should be. Further, Catholic teaching's consistent life ethic requires a grasp of the whole picture along with a commitment to being responsible for how changes to one element affect all the others.

The Lack of Family Orientation

We have already described Catholic Social teaching's insistence on viewing adolescents within the context of their families. The importance of such a view is borne out by the experience of health care workers and by scholarly research. Health care professionals and researchers are increasingly aware that the most efficient and effective health delivery system for Americans is a family-centered system (Consortium of Family Organizations, 1992; Snyder & Ooms, 1992; Children's Defense Fund, 1992; Campbell & Treat, 1990; Doherty & McCubbin, 1985). This conclusion relies heavily on research cited above which shows the powerful influence of the family on the health behaviors and illnesses of family members as well as the effects of family members' health, illness, and disabilities on family functioning (Consortium of Family Organizations, 1992; Campbell & Treat, 1990; Doherty & Campbell, 1988). Recent psychoanalytic understandings of adolescence, furthermore, indicate that adolescence is characterized by a time of renegotiation of parent-child relationships; such renegotiations inherently involve the parents as well as the individual young person (Steinberg, 1990).

Unfortunately, most health care services are oriented toward the individual patient; relatively few service delivery systems are family-oriented. According to Doherty and Campbell (1988), most medical facilities practice a minimum level of family involvement. At most medical schools, university hospitals, and tertiary care medical centers, the:

> . . . family is not regarded as a conscious object of attention and concern for clinicians, except insofar as practical and legal reasons require contact with the family. The individual patient is the sole focus of attention, and often the focus is only on the patient's disease process. (Doherty & Campbell, 1988: 134)

Rarely is there a free exchange even of "medical" information or a collaboration among adolescent patients, their parents, and their physicians. Even more rare is an understanding of the family's role in the ongoing health of the adolescent, the role of the adolescent in the health of other family members, or the need for collaboration between medical professionals and the adolescent and his or her family.

The experience of drug and alcohol abuse programs indicates that changing the behavior of adolescents alone is not sufficient to bring about lasting changes in their health-compromising behaviors (Snyder & Ooms, 1992). More than occasional information from adults is needed because often problems are centered in the family. As Wendy Snyder and Theodora Ooms point out:

> (p)rofessionals began to suspect that treatment needed to include family members in order to address their own concerns and help them recognize how their own actions might be maintaining the adolescent's problem behaviors, even as they aspired to change them. The family could then be mobilized as a resource in support of stable behavior change. (1992: 3)

Characteristics of Health Care Services

Other important barriers to service delivery to adolescents include the convenience of the facility, its ambience, and the quality of the staff/teen communication. The physical setting and decor of the waiting room are important to some teens. Pediatricians who have an adolescent practice need to have reading materials appropriate to teenagers as well as toys for waiting toddlers and young children. Similarly, family practitioners, obstetricians and other specialists with adolescent clientele should be aware of the atmosphere created by providing only "adult" reading material; pamphlets concerning the need for regular cancer screening after age 40 or on the dangers of osteoporosis will be unlikely to make any 16-year-old feel that the facilities are appropriate for her.

Like other patients, teens appreciate prompt and appropriate treatment. Adolescents seem to be particularly subject to discouragement if they experience a long delay in phone access to physicians for advice. Long waits before getting an appointment or a holdup before receiving treatment also may discourage adolescent involvement in their own health.

The embarrassment adolescents may experience in regard to obtaining health care lessen the likelihood of their seeking health care. (Long, 1985; Rogers & Elliott, 1989). Additionally, adolescents often don't use health care facilities because they fear condescension, lecturing, or moral preaching from the staff (Kisker, 1985; Vernon & Seymore, 1987). Similarly, adolescents' perceptions of community clinics may limit their willingness to visit such facilities. While those who have visited clinics rate them favorably, those who have yet to visit them are likely to see clinics as "dirty places" serving "undesirables" (Kisker, 1985).

An adolescent's experience in a health care facility will likely affect his or her willingness to utilize formal health care in the future. A strong determinant of that experience is the adolescent's interaction with clinic personnel. Some research points out several factors common to adolescents that make such interactions potentially problematic (Long, 1985). Adolescents are sometimes skeptical about adults and almost all health care providers are adults. As teens search for autonomy, some are especially sensitive to adult domination; treatment and recommendations by health care workers may be interpreted as domination rather than aid. Similarly, adolescents have a tendency to be more idealistic than their health-care providers. Such idealism may result in frustration on the part of the adolescent, physician or counselor. Furthermore, the adolescents may sense feelings of discomfort or ambivalence in the care provider, especially during their discussion of sexuality-related issues (Long, 1985).

Adolescents and their families may also be unaware of existing services. Effective service delivery to teens involves not only the provision of health care services but promoting these services in areas where adolescents and their families are likely to find out about them (DuRant, 1991; U. S. Congress, Office of Technology Assessment, 1991a).

Cultural Barriers to the Use of Health Care Services

Cultural variations clearly influence adolescents' access to medical services, the likelihood that they will seek medical treatment, the quality and effectiveness of the treatment they will receive, and the chances that they will receive care at all. Some minority families find it hard to access appropriate health care services because of language or reading difficulties; a substantial portion of minority youth and their families do not have English as their primary language and many others are functionally illiterate. For many of those whose primary language is Spanish, for instance, the lack of health care personnel translates into real inconveniences such as longer waiting times before appointments with one of the few American physicians who is fluent in both Spanish and English (Andersen, Giachello, & Aday, 1986). Some ethnic minority groups are comprised largely of relatively recent immigrants; a few such as the Hmong have moved directly from a preliterate society to a modern high-technology society, resulting in a full range of acculturation difficulties. For these adolescents and their families, the task of accessing appropriate health care services is often overwhelming. Furthermore, because poverty and low incomes are more common among minority groups than among White, non-Latino populations, the cost of health care persuades some families to avoid even seeking care except in emergency situations.

Some minority adolescents attribute their under-utilization of health care services to cultural biases on the part of the health care professionals. Black, Latino, Native Americans, and many other ethnic minorities are underrepresented in professional health care positions (Airhihenbuwa, 1989; Association of American Medical Colleges, 1993). For example, in the 1992-93 school year only 7.8% of medical school applicants were Black, .5% Native American, 1.9% Mexican American or Chicano, and .6% Puerto Rican residents of the mainland U.S. (Association of American Medical Colleges, 1993: 37).

Medical service providers are best attuned to the dominant culture in this country: that of middle-class Caucasians of European descent. Cultural assumptions concerning what constitutes appropriate behaviors, what constitutes health and well-being, and how anger, depression, and guilt are expressed vary from group to group and are all tied to the chances of receiving appropriate medical care. Variations in affective expression are often culturally based; what is an appropriate expression of emotion for a

Vietnamese American is very different from what is considered appropriate in a White family with an Italian heritage. Coping mechanisms differ from one subculture to another as do the very nature of family relationships, the nature of authority, interpersonal competence, and feelings of self-worth. Such differences translate into different abilities, needs, and chances to access medical care in this country. These variations in cultural assumptions and behaviors often compound any difficulties minority groups might have accessing needed medical services due to increased chances of being poor, living in under-served areas, and being subject to the vagaries of racism.

Some relatively minor cultural differences may translate into serious medical misdiagnoses. Allen and Majidi-Ahi, for instance, point out that differences in communication styles may make it more probable that psychologists and counselors will make a misdiagnosis:

> Blacks often converse among themselves while engaging in another activity. It is understood within the group that one can participate in the conversation without needing to maintain constant eye contact. However, among clinicians, avoidance of eye contact is an important criterion of relatedness. Consequently, clinicians who work with Black children must consider other indexes of social relatedness before concluding that a Black child has problems in social development because of "poor" eye contact. (1990: 162)

For some ethnic and racial minorities, cultural differences affect the health of the young people in terms of a "culture clash" with the dominant values and practices. Puerto Rican parents on the mainland, for instance, often have difficulty maintaining control over the behaviors of their adolescent children. Researchers point out, however, that these families often lack cultural supports for increasing autonomy among young people:

> First-generation parents operate within a framework that considers offspring to be children, regardless of age or responsibilities, until they become adults. Adulthood is usually marked by marriage or leaving home, whichever comes first. Viewed as children, adolescents are expected to subordinate their views and interests to those of the parents, to show respect, and to follow the guidelines of behavior and etiquette that the parents provide . . . Puerto Rican adolescents reared in the United States and exposed to its socializing influences begin to expect and demand an "adolescence," with all its freedoms. This is an especially stressful demand to make for female Puerto Rican adolescents, whose requests are viewed within the cultural double standard that encourages sexual activity and increased freedom for the males and abstinence and overprotectiveness of the females. (Inclan & Herron, 1990: 262)

Given this clash of values, adolescents are more likely to exaggerate their health-compromising behaviors in order to express their independence and autonomy.

Similarly, some cultural differences necessitate different treatments and differences in the structure of health-care delivery systems. This is the case, for example, for Native American adolescents whose cultures generally emphasize interdependence and community, and the ethic of sharing everything with others, while allowing a relatively high degree of autonomy at a young age. Medical services which emphasize the adolescent as an individual--the isolated recipient of a pathogen or single unhealthy behavior--are unlikely to be well received. Conversely, those facilities that undermine the decision-making prerogatives accorded these teenagers by their parents are likely to be viewed as an anathema by these young people and their families (LaFromboise & Low, 1990).

Those health care professionals who treat youth of various ethnic and racial groups are faced with the task of developing sensitivity to a number of different cultural assumptions (Allen & Majidi-Ahi, 1990; Huang & Gibbs, 1990; Ramirez, 1990). The vast cultural differences between ethnic groups within broader racial categories often complicate this process. An Asian doctor of Chinese heritage, for instance, may know relatively little about relevant cultural assumptions of Vietnamese immigrants (Liu & Yu, 1985). Similarly, the experiences of middle-class Black physicians do not necessarily prepare them to recognize the impact of culture on Black adolescents from Jamaica or Haiti or Africa or Cuba, or, for that matter, an inner-city ghetto.

Financial Barriers to Adolescent Health Care

A very serious barrier to using available services is lack of health insurance and limitations in coverage among at-risk adolescents and their families. The decision to seek health care is more often driven by the extent to which the treatment is seen as affordable by the adolescents and their parents rather than by the perceived "need" of care or treatment (Cromer, 1992). In 1988, 15% of all adolescents were without public or private health insurance (U.S. Congress, Office of Technology Assessment, 1991c). Most of the poor adolescents who were insured received coverage through Medicaid but more than 30% of adolescents with family incomes below the poverty line were without any insurance (Kronick, 1989; U.S. Congress, Office of Technology Assessment, 1991c).

Monheit and Cunningham (1992) point out that differences in insurance status among teens translate directly into differences in access to a usual source of health care as well as differences in the likelihood that the young people will obtain particular medical services.[47] Figure 4.3 illustrates some of these differences. For example, while nearly three quarters of the teens who were privately insured during 1987 saw a physician during that year, only about 46% of those who had neither private nor public health insurance had contact with a doctor. Similarly, about 60% of those with private health insurance received dental services during 1987 while less than 19% of those without insurance visited a dentist.

Even among those who are covered by health insurance, policies stipulate which types of medical services are covered and which are not. While private, employment-based, health insurance policies typically protect against the major costs of hospital and physician-provided services for those with acute illness, many other types of health care are not covered by these policies (U.S. Congress, Office of Technology Assessment, 1991c: 84). According to surveys conducted by the Health Insurance Association of America (HIAA) and the Bureau of Labor Statistics, however, preventatie diagnostic care is covered for only about 69% of those with suc private group insurance[48] (U.S. Congress, Office of Technology Assessment 1991c). Similarly, rouine physical exams were covered by only 28% of the policies, immunizations by only 29% of the policies, and general dental Assessment, 1991c). In some cases, specific conditions are excluded from coverage for teenagers; in other cases, specific conditions are provided only limited coverage. Most notable, for example, is a pattern of exclusion for the cost of maternity-related services for adolescent daughters of privately insured parents (U.S. Congress, Office of Technology Assessment, 1991c). Furthermore, mental health care coverage is almost always more limited than coverage for "physical" ailments (Cromer, 1992). For instance, only 28% of policies cover the costs of hospitalization for detoxification[49] the

---

[47] These differences are probably most pronounced for conditions that are not seen as acute emergencies by service providers. Among even the most destitute, emergency care is generally available regardless of their family's ability to pay.

[48] These surveys were both done in 1988. The HIAA surveyed 1,665 randomly selected employers offering coverage to their employees. It excluded those who obtain their own insurance and Federal employees. The survey conduced by the Bureau of Labor Statistics is based on a sample of 1,922 nonfarm organizations employing more than 100 employees (Office of Technology Assessment, 1991c: 84-85).

[49] Detoxification involves medical supervision of the use of medication to reduce or eliminate the effects of substance abuse (Office of Technology Assessment, 1991c: 90).

FIGURE 4.3:   Percent of 13- to 17-Year-Olds with Contact with
Medical Services During 1987 by Insurance Status

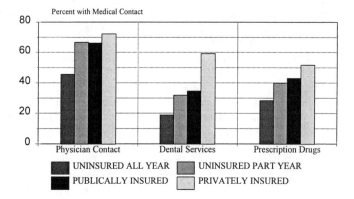

SOURCE: Adapted from Monheit & Cunningham, 1992, *The Future of*
Children: U.S. Health Care for Childen, Tables A2, A4, and A5 pp.
166-167. Data were collected by the Agency for Health Care Policy
and Research, 1987 National Medical Expenditure Survey.

same way they would injuries sustained from a car accident (U.S. Congress,
Office of Technology Assessment, 1991c: 90). Given the prevalence of
social morbidities among the adolescent population, such benefit
restrictions are clearly problematic.
care by only 37% of the policies (U.S. Congress, Office of Technology

For those with public insurance the financial obstacles to health care are
even more of a deterrent. Eligibility requirements, services offered,
utilization limits, and provider payment policies all vary widely from state
to state. In 1989, Congress began to require states to periodically screen
Medicaid-eligible adolescents for illnesses, abnormalities, or treatable
conditions and cover their treatment through the Early Periodic Screening,
Diagnosis, and Treatment (EPSDT) program (Children's Defense Fund,
1990; U.S. Congress, Office of Technology Assessment, 1991a). However,
if the U.S. is going to rely on the current Medicaid system to provide
adequate medical care to the poor, states must expand Medicaid eligibility
to all poor adolescents and increase the number of Medicaid providers.
Hopefully, a large portion of the financial barriers to adolescent health care

delivery will be remedied by the restructuring of the health care systems in the United States during the next few years.

CHAPTER 5

ISSUES IN ADOLESCENT SERVICE DELIVERY

While there is little debate concerning the propriety of eliminating these barriers to efficient and adequate health-care services, there are a number of issues which surround the delivery of adolescent health care that raise complicated ethical and moral choices for practitioners and for society as a whole. Three of these issues are discussed here: the prevention and treatment of social morbidities; the appropriate role for the family in the delivery of health care to adolescents; and the role of schools in health treatment and education.

TREATMENT AND PREVENTION OF SOCIAL MORBIDITIES

Effective health care delivery to adolescents warrants a perspective that acknowledges the complexity of the relationship among adolescents' behaviors, physiology, social situations, and their health status. Such a multidimensional bio-psychosocial perspective seems likely to prove useful for developing prevention and treatment strategies, but presupposes an understanding of the complex nature of the causes and consequences of social morbidities.

Traditionally, most health-compromising behaviors have been defined somewhat superficially. These risky behaviors have been viewed by some as deviant, sinful, or criminal activities rather than in any way biological or social-psychological. Their ties to the developmental stages of adolescence have generally been ignored. The physical and emotional sequelae of these behaviors have often been seen as appropriate punishment for the teens' activities: just rewards for young people "sowing their wild oats."

Yet both the causes and the results of many risky behaviors have ties to adolescents' physiology and the social pressures that characterize this period of life. Adolescents' likely participation in these health-compromising behaviors is tied to their physical and mental development. It is typical of adolescents to push the limits of parental control, experiment with risky activities, and maintain a belief in their own immortality:

> During the adolescent years, individuals typically will experiment with a wide range of behaviors and life-style patterns. This experimentation is all part of the natural process of separating from parents, developing a sense of autonomy and independence, establishing a personal identity, and acquiring the skills necessary for functioning effectively in the adult world. (Schinke, Botvin, & Orlandi, 1991: 11)

Adolescents, precisely because of their incomplete cognitive development and their consistent belief in their own invulnerability, frequently exhibit a remarkable absence of concern about the possible adverse consequences of their health-compromising behaviors (Elkind, 1992; Schinke, Botvin, & Orlandi, 1991). From this perspective, risk-taking is associated with all of the changes and uncertainties of adolescence; it is an expected developmental condition of adolescence just as much as are rapid growth, sexual maturation, and the onset of acne.

Similarly, the consequences of the social morbidities are biological as well as social-psychological. Since adolescents' exposure to violence and participation in violent activities are causing many injuries and deaths, it is reasonable to view *violence* itself as a *pathogen* and treat violent teens and their victims as patients rather than simply as criminals. Since early sexual activity promotes the spread of STD's with serious biological and social consequences, and also promotes early undesired pregnancies, births, and abortions, one could logically view early sexual activity as a truly *medical* problem as well as an indication of moral weakness. Since substance and alcohol abuse among adolescents have serious *medical* consequences including chemical addiction, brain damage, and death, society and its health care practitioners could recognize the use and abuse of illicit drugs and alcohol by adolescents as medical problems as well as delinquent behaviors chosen by many teenagers.

When social morbidities are viewed from such a perspective, the focus shifts away from threats and punishment and toward treatment and prevention. If social morbidities are viewed primarily as deviant, sinful, or criminal activities, then the focus of treatment is on the cessation of immoral and risky behaviors precisely because they are illegal, immoral or bad. Treatment is equated largely with punishment--making the enjoyment of the behavior not worth its presumed risk to the participant. A multidimensional perspective which includes the medical and societal roots of these conditions would logically alter the emphasis of the treatment of social morbidities toward their avoidance because it is clear to the adolescents that, while the behaviors are "reasonable" responses to the challenges and conditions they face, these same behaviors pose a very real physical threat to their health and well-being. An understanding that these health-compromising behaviors have both social roots and physical ramifications would lead directly to the treatment of the illnesses' likely concomitancies.

It appears that in the case of adolescent violence, early sexual activity, and adolescent substance abuse the prevention of these behaviors through punitive measures has not been very effective. Despite the argument that alcohol abuse by adolescents is "sinful" or "delinquent" or "criminal," teenagers continue to drink, consume alcohol at earlier and earlier ages, and continue to die in alcohol-related accidents. Physical violence is clearly defined as a criminal activity--its treatment generally punitive--yet the use of physical violence by adolescents and against adolescents continues unabated in the United States. Similarly, early sexual activity--especially when it results in a pregnancy--is defined as "delinquent," "morally wrong," and in some cases "criminal," yet increasing numbers of American adolescents initiate sexual activity while they are very young. Perhaps the "Just Say No" campaigns of the 1980's were less effective than they might have been because they did not expressly acknowledge either the social or the biological roots of these risky behaviors.[50]

The definition of risky, health-compromising behaviors away from the realm of deviance and crime toward a more bio-psychosocial perspective carries with it, however, a number of serious implications (Conrad & Schneider, 1980; Kittrie, 1971; Szasz, 1961). Advocating such a change is not morally neutral; divestment of the criminal justice system tends to legitimate intervention by other professionals even in areas where they have no track record of success. Such a redefinition of behaviors implies that risk-taking behaviors cannot be attributed exclusively to the moral weakness of the adolescent. If violence, substance abuse, and early sexual activity are bio-psychosocial conditions--illnesses of sorts with social roots--then their "cures" are unlikely to be found in punishment, criminalization, or incarceration. Bio-psychosocial conditions call for social and medical interventions.

---

[50] According to an analysis by Victor Strasburger, the "Just Say No" campaigns against drug and alcohol use were not well suited to adolescent audiences because the slogan says *what* to do rather than *why* one should do it or *how* one should go about it (1989).

A more detailed analysis of the issues involved in this debate for three important social morbidities follows.

Understanding Violence as a Multidimensional Problem

This perspective suggests that those who provide health care services to adolescents should consider both the *exposure to* violence and *use of* violence as multidimensional problems. While violence by and against adolescents is generally both immoral and criminal, the other dimensions of violence should be seen as well. The biological ties to violence are logically clear: violence is closely tied to injury, mutilation, and death. Its social and psychological roots are also clear; violence is clearly a learned behavior. Those adolescents who experience violence in their homes and neighborhoods are less likely to find non-violent ways of dealing with stress, anger, and external threats. The use of violence against adolescents results in a large proportion of the injuries and deaths suffered by this age group. Violence against oneself is suicidal behavior. The use of violence all too often results in the injury or death of the aggressor.

If violence is defined as a bio-psychosocial condition, the *prevention* of violence and violent behavior becomes a logical focus of health care for adolescents. Instead of simply criminals and victims--the guilty and the innocent--more emphasis is placed on the individuals as patients: the injured, the sick, and the susceptible (Trafford, 1992). The reduction in the underlying social causes of violence (poverty and hopelessness) and in the availability of the primary tools of violence (guns) becomes a reasonable focus for practitioners (Adelson, 1992; Anderson, 1995).

The American Medical Association has worked in recent years to redefine violence as a "medical" problem. Then Surgeon General Antonia C. Novello has acknowledged this perspective:

> Just as we health professionals have done for other health problems, we have a clear duty to take a leadership role in the antiviolence movement. We must press for changes in economic conditions and insist on expanded access to health care.
>
> . . . (T)he prevention of violence by using public health methods in our communities is as much our responsibility as is the treatment of its victims. (Novello, Shosky, & Froehlke, 1992: 3007)

Similarly, the Centers for Disease Control and Prevention has recently funded three multi-million dollar research grants which are founded on the premise that youth violence is a preventable problem. "Kids are killing kids and we think it's a fact of life in this country," explained a spokesperson for this public health agency. "But people thought smallpox was a fact of life too, and it's been eradicated from the face of the Earth" (Associated Press, *Dayton Daily News*, July 14, 1993: 4A). The programs involve teaching conflict resolution and peer mediation skills, mentoring teens by professionals. The public health officials of the Centers for Disease Control and Prevention have also worked to reduce the availability of handguns in much the same way as they might seek the elimination of more traditional pathogens (Associated Press, *Dayton Daily News*, 1993; Trafford, 1992).

Early Sexual Activity as a Multidimensional Problem

Similar insights can be gathered if one considers early sexual activity from a multidimensional perspective. While sexual activity outside of marriage is commonplace in our society, it runs directly contrary to Catholic moral teaching along a number of fronts. Such behavior rarely shows respect for the dignity of the individuals involved; often it results in their degradation rather than affirmation. The prevalence of such unchaste relationships can be seen as a reflection of the "divorce culture" rather than upholding the importance of marriage and the family (Hackstaff, 1994).

Viewing early sexual activity as a bio-psychosocial problem places the focus of analysis squarely on the health-compromising behavior. All adolescents who engage in early sexual activity are putting themselves at risk for numerous difficulties.[51] They significantly increase their likelihood of contracting a number of serious diseases, including AIDS. They are subject to a very real risk of early parenthood, and the young women are subject to the multiple complications of pregnancy and abortion. This perspective underscores the fact that such behaviors pose real risks to *both* young women and men. Traditional double-standard arguments that early sexual activity is acceptable (or even desirable) for males but unacceptable for females are refuted by the logic of this perspective.

---

[51] It is important to note that many of the adolescents who are defined as "sexually active" report that they have been subjected to unwanted sexual contact by a boyfriend, friend, first date, or other adult. Small and Kerns, for instance, report that about 20% of female adolescents in their study of 1,149 teenagers in grades 7, 9, and 11 had been subjected to some sort of forced sexual contact during the year previous to the study (1993: 941). Approximately 8% of those surveyed reported that they were *forced* to have sexual intercourse during the previous year (Small & Kerns, 1993: 946).

> Anna was 16 when she first visited this clinic because of recurrent
> pain in the groin. She has been sexually active since she was 13 and
> reports only sporadic use of condoms. While her pregnancy test was
> negative, the examination and culture did reveal an infection. In
> addition to receiving medication , she was counseled concerning the
> damaging effects of repeated STD infections, the possible effects of
> STD's on any subsequent pregnancy, and the advantages of avoiding
> further infection through sexual contact.

SOURCE: Kathleen Vesha, RN and Roseann Schoenbachler, RN, Columbus
Children's Hospital Teen Clinic, Columbus, OH, correspondence
with the authors, July 3, 1995.

This perspective views the contracting of a sexually transmitted disease
or an unanticipated pregnancy as a *symptom* of this risky behavior. The
pivotal problem is not pregnancy prevention or avoidance of gonorrhea, but
the early sexual activity itself. Furthermore, any program which seeks to
alleviate only the presenting symptoms cannot be expected to "cure" the
adolescent. Seeing early sexual activity as the central problem shifts
attention from the treatment of symptoms to the underlying psychological,
cultural, and biological conditions which foster the initiation and
continuation of sexual activity among adolescents.

It also implies an understanding that sexual activity does not occur in a
social vacuum. There are very real social (and physical) pressures which
make early sexual activity attractive to many young people. It is not
surprising that the argument that it is "wrong" to have nonmarital sex
continues to fall on deaf ears in a culture which consistently promotes sex
as a vehicle for happiness, popularity, and power. The popular media have
consistently glorified sexual activity, while the costs associated with an
undesired pregnancy or the contraction of a STD are rarely spelled out.
For many, the risks of early sexual activity appear relatively minor in
comparison with the constant and immediate threats associated with
poverty and its concomitant violence. For others, the risk of social
rejection or the desire for independence and autonomy are more
threatening and immediate than the risks they perceive to be associated
with their own sexual activity. An effective response to adolescent sexual
activity presupposes a perspective that acknowledges the immense social
pressures facing today's youth to become sexually active.

Donna came with her mother to the prenatal clinic for her first appointment. They appeared affluent and were from a wealthy suburb. As I began to talk with Donna about her plans for the baby, her mother said , "Oh, we're not keeping this baby." Donna responded with, "Yes we are!" That is when the battle lines were formed. Her mother made it very clear that there was no way that she would be allowed to bring the baby home. As the months went by, support was given to both Donna and her mother, but neither one would give in even a little bit. Donna is an example of a determined young woman. She went into foster care at the end of her pregnancy and lived there for a number of months with her baby, in a crowded house. This was quite a change in lifestyle from what she had been used to. Eventually, Donna's mother did eventually let them both move back home and she now speaks lovingly of her grandson.

During the fall of her senior year, Sherise managed to deny her pregnancy despite nausea and weight gain. Neither she nor her mother ever questioned her changing condition until she woke up one night feeling that she had a stomach flu. After watching T.V. for a while, she screamed and delivered a healthy 8 pound daughter on the living room floor. When her mother woke up, she passed out at the sight. It was an adjustement for the family, but they all welcomed this baby.

Carolyn came from a very difficult home. She chose to move out to avoid her mother's various addictions as well as her abusive boyfriends. Chronically absent from school, Carolyn eventually dropped out and became quite depressed. Being pregnant at 15 compounded her problems. During the first year of her son's life she lived in eight different apartments and never had a bed of her own. Both she and the baby suffered from recurrent sore throats and ear aches and nutritional deficiencies. The baby's 23 year old father is unable and unwilling to provide any help to either his son or his young mother.

SOURCE: Patty Martin, R.N., Miami Valley Hospital, correspondence with Joan McGuinness Wagner, June 22, 1995.

Substance and Alcohol Abuse as a Multidimensional Problem

Like nonmarital sexual activity, the abuse of alcohol and drugs is common throughout American society. The popularity of alcohol in this country is reflected in its industry's multi-million dollar presence; its use is promoted in the printed and electronic media. Though common, the abuse of alcohol and other drugs tends to thwart authentic human development, often causes serious problems within families, and debases rather than dignifies individual persons. Thus the abuse of drugs and alcohol by adults as well as adolescents often can be seen as a breach of Catholic teaching.

It is equally easy to see the biological effects of alcohol and substance abuse even if the analysis of this adolescent health-compromising behavior is limited to pharmacological ramifications. The focus of treatment is reducing the negative side-effects of their use. If these behaviors are viewed solely as indications of moral weakness or a propensity toward criminality, then punishment is the logical "cure" for this problem. Viewing these behaviors as bio-psychosocial health problems--as well as behavior that undermines authentic human development--shifts the emphasis to the elimination of a vast array of conditions that pressure some adolescents to begin using illicit substances, tobacco, or alcohol. If drug abuse is not viewed solely as "bad" behavior, its social and developmental precursors can be addressed along with its medical and psychological concomitancies.

PARENTAL INVOLVEMENT AND ADOLESCENT AUTONOMY

Another major issue facing the adolescent health care system is finding the appropriate level of family involvement for young people who are in the process of establishing the autonomy accorded adults in our society (Grochowski & Bach, 1994). Health care issues pertaining to parental involvement and adolescent autonomy are revealed in questions surrounding confidentiality, parental notification, and parental consent. Catholic teaching emphasizes the role of parents as educators and guides for their children. This emphasis, and its more secular counterparts, can be seen in existent policies and programs relating to teen health. In many religious and secular health care systems, parents are presumed to be better able than their children to understand the sequelae of a given condition and its treatment. They are assumed to have the best interests of their child in mind when they make treatment decisions in consultation with the health practitioners. Furthermore, it is generally the parents who are responsible for the financial burdens of medical care for their children; they should therefore have a say in the appropriateness of the treatment.

Parental responsibility?

Sometimes you just want to shake your head. . . A few months ago, for example, the nicest young man and his friend came into the E.R. It seems his mother was too busy to come in, so another friend dropped them off. I think the story was that the mother had a paper to write or a class to teach the next day. Her 14- year- old son had just taken most of a bottle of Tylenol and had confided to his friend that he didn't want to live anymore. Fortunately , the friend was forceful enough to talk the Mom into paying for a taxi for him. It wouldn't have been easy; the mother was extremely annoyed that she was required to come to the hospital to sign the Consent to Treat forms. She signed the papers and gave him her cash card so that he could get taxi money from the machine in the lobby. What else could she do? Anyway we pumped his stomach, got him stablized, had him speak with a counselor, and watched him call a cab and leave a few hours later.

SOURCE: Barbara Richardson, R.N., Emergency Room, Children's Medical Center, Dayton, OH, conversation with the author, April, 1996.

Yet in practice, determinations of the most appropriate role for adolescents and their families to play in health care decisions are often difficult. Since adolescents pass through different stages in the process of maturing, not all 19-year-olds are necessarily capable of "adult" reasoning and not all 16-year-olds are too immature to be granted a good deal of autonomy. Similarly, some parents are better able than others to make the decisions which truly reflect the best interests of their teenagers. Some parents, most adolescents, and some medical professionals lack an understanding of the many relevant medical, psychosocial, and ethical issues that will form the foundation upon which rational decisions about medical care should be based. When parents are in fact limited by their knowledge and ability to discern what is in the best interests of their offspring, mandated parental or family involvement sometimes becomes problematic.

There is some evidence to suggest that at times the laudable goal of family involvement may serve as a significant barrier to the efficient delivery of health care services to adolescents (Ambuel & Rappaport, 1992). Even the *perception* that services will not be provided confidentially is enough to hinder some teens from seeking medical care. Adolescents who do not want their parents to be informed of their desire or need for certain health care services may find parental consent policies a cogent barrier to their health care. Some of these teens then avoid seeking treatment until the ailment worsens or goes away. In these cases, a lack of confidentiality is counter-productive to the quality and timeliness of medical treatment. A parental consent policy, or the teens' perceptions of such a requirement, is a barrier to the efficient delivery of health care services for some adolescents.

Some attempts to resolve the issues of confidentiality and parental consent for health care services--issues of authority--have been made by the courts. In most cases, the authority for health care decisions for adolescent patients resides squarely in the parents' lap until their son or daughter reaches the age of majority. The government generally requires parental consent for surgical and medical care for two main reasons. First, it is presumed that adolescents lack the capacity to make sound judgments about their own health. A good deal of empirical research, however, refutes this argument. These data suggest that adolescents--especially older ones--are more competent to make decisions than is usually legally assumed (Ambuel, 1990; Ambuel & Rappaport, 1992; Rodman, Lewis, & Griffith, 1984; Melton, 1983).

The second reason government generally requires parental consent for medical treatment is so the state can encourage family involvement in the minors' lives (U.S. Congress, Office of Technology Assessment, 1991c: 123). Deeply embedded in Anglo-American law as well as the Judeo-Christian tradition is the belief:

> that the parental consent requirement *promotes family autonomy and privacy and promotes parental authority and control of minor children.* Family autonomy and parental authority, in turn, are often viewed as fostering the stability and cohesiveness of the family as an institution and of individual family units. (emphasis in the original {U.S. Congress, Office of Technology Assessment, 1991c: 125})

Legally and ethically, there are a number of "exceptions" to the parental consent rules. These exceptions include abused and neglected adolescents under court supervision; those who are legally emancipated, particularly mature, or independent; health emergencies; and adolescents with specific health problems such as drug or alcohol abuse, mental illness treatment, and services related to sexual activity (U.S. Congress, Office of Technology

Assessment, 1991c). The logic of these exceptions is that in some cases--the proportion of cases is hotly debated--adolescents receive more timely and appropriate care *without* the involvement of their families.

The extent to which parental consent requirements serve to bolster family autonomy and stability is unknown; conversely, the extent to which parental consent requirements are seen by some adolescents as a barrier to health care services has been documented only in the case of the delivery of services related to sexual activity. Some of these data suggest that a sizeable portion of sexually active adolescents will postpone requesting contraceptive services or travel to other jurisdictions if they believe that their parents will necessarily be told of their request (Zabin & Clark, 1981; Chamie, Eisman, Forrest, Orr, & Torres, 1982; Cartoof & Klerman, 1986; Blum, Resnick, & Stark, 1987).

Other research, however, indicates that enactment of parental notification laws does not necessarily result in treatment avoidance or migration. The authors of an investigation of the impact of a parental notification law in Minnesota report that it was associated with declines in abortion rates among young women aged 15 to 17 (Rogers, Boruch, Stoms, & DeMoya, 1991).[52] These data also indicate that, at least initially, enactment of this law facilitated pregnancy avoidance among adolescent women under 17. Furthermore, the authors of this study found no indications that the law resulted in treatment avoidance; they did not find an increase in late abortions among these young people (Rogers, Boruch, Stoms, & DeMoya, 1991).

Medical service providers appear somewhat ambivalent about legally required parental consent as well as about the assumption that patient confidentiality can be ethically extended to teenage patients (Novack, Detering, Arnold, Forrow, Ladinsky, & Pezzullo, 1989). Perhaps in part because parental consent facilitates compensation for their services, some health care providers support the parental consent laws (Cromer, 1992; U.S. Congress, Office of Technology Assessment, 1991c: 123). Those physicians who treat many adolescents, however, are less likely to see parental consent as being more important than patient confidentiality for their clients. A survey of physicians who are members of the Society for

---

[52]   The authors explain the discrepancies in their findings with those of Cartoof and Klerman (1986) by pointing out that minors in Massachusetts face very different conditions from those in Minnesota. They point out that "Minnesota is a unique state with a low minority population and a low pregnancy rate even before parental notice." Furthermore, in comparison to the youth of Massachusetts, those in Minnesota are geographically isolated and are not easily able to migrate to surrounding states without similar legislation to obtain abortions (Rogers, Boruch, Stoms, & DeMoya, 1991).

Adolescent Medicine, for example, indicates that 75% believe patient confidentiality should take precedence over parental authority (Lovett & Wald, 1985).

THE ROLE OF SCHOOLS IN HEALTH TREATMENT AND EDUCATION

A closely related issue involves the role of schools in health treatment and education. Some argue that schools are usurping the place of parents in adolescent lives. Others see schools as having the most direct access to students who often lack adequate support and direction from their parents. Some, perhaps because they do not see the bio-psychosocial roots of the adolescents' health-compromising behaviors, believe that health education in schools should be limited to physiology or personal hygiene. Discussions surrounding the role of schools in adolescent health care focus on the appropriateness of providing comprehensive health care services within schools and the content and timing of health-related curricula.

School-Based or School-Linked Health Clinics

Because schools offer the unique opportunity to reach a large portion of adolescents in a particular vicinity, they have become a common site for the treatment of some adolescent health problems. Usually, the treatment offered to adolescents in schools is rather minimal. School nurses generally offer first aid and some preventative screenings but have neither the resources nor the authority to provide much more.

School-based and school-linked health centers differ from traditional in-school medical services in a number of ways. First, they have the authority and mandate to provide more comprehensive health care services to the students. Most have the authority to prescribe medications. Unlike traditional school medical services, school-based centers are staffed by physicians and other professionals such as nutritionists, dentists, psychologists and social workers. Since such a mandate requires a substantial increase in resources, most school-based facilities are funded by organizations and groups that are not accountable directly to the board of education. Hospitals, public health departments, private foundations, and corporations have all funded school-based clinics (Dryfoos, 1988; Glasow, 1988; Kirby, Waszak, & Ziegler, 1989; Lear, 1992; Riessman, 1991). Such funding situations make issues of accountability--authority and responsibility for the health and well-being of the teens--even more complex than in traditional health care delivery settings.

Some argue that, because the school systems are not directly accountable for the services provided on their premises, school-based health clinics may easily undermine parental authority. Adolescent health clinics generally address the question of parental authority by requiring some sort of parental consent form. Some school-based health clinics require a signed consent form for each visit, some ask for parental consent for each type of service, others present a "blanket" consent for treatment for the entire school year, and still others use a check-off list requesting parents to mark off those services which are unacceptable for their children. All adolescent clinics which access government funds from Title X or Title XX require some form of parental consent; the effectiveness of such consent is a matter of debate. School-based health clinics, like all other private health service providers, are subject to local, state, and federal statutes concerning confidentiality and parental access to medical files.

In some areas, school-based or school-linked health clinics represent a costly duplication of services, but in others they provide the most direct and consistent contact with a sizeable portion of an otherwise difficult-to-reach population. According to the Center for Population Options, many of the adolescents using school-based health clinics do not have other adequate sources of health care:

> Approximately half of all students and three-fifths of elementary and junior high/middle school students using school-based and school-linked clinics do not have access to other sources of health care. In some clinics, the proportion of teens without access to other health care approaches 100 percent. Less than 20 percent of clinic users are covered by private insurance or health maintenance organizations; nearly 40 percent are completely uninsured. (Riessman, 1991:1)

Most of the school-based health clinics are built in low-income areas where access to health care is severely limited by both lack of insurance coverage and a lack of transportation to other facilities.

In those areas where the adolescents are under-served, much of the literature from Catholic authors suggests that the site of the clinic is less important than the content of the treatment programs involved. In their *Statement on School-Based Clinics,* for example, the Bishops of the United States state:

> School-based health clinics that clearly separate themselves from the agenda of contraceptive advocates may provide part of an effective response to the health needs of young people. (1987:439)

Provided the programs do not usurp parental authority, dispense contraceptives, or in any way suggest to adolescents that sexual activity and abortion are sanctioned, school-based or school-linked health care centers provide a good opportunity to meet at least some of the health care needs of adolescents.

Because many school-based clinics were started in reaction to a need to address the high rate of adolescent pregnancies, by groups which view artificial means of birth control as preferable to teenage pregnancy and parenting, school-based health clinics are sometimes equated with birth-control clinics (Glasow, 1988). According to Lear's analysis of the 58,000 visits to school-based health centers during the 1989-1990 school year, 12% concerned reproductive health or sexually transmitted diseases (Lear, 1992: 900). Survey results of school-based clinics indicate that many school-based health clinics do not dispense or prescribe contraceptives of any sort on (Kirby, Waszak, & Ziegler, 1989). More recent data[53] indicate that about 40% of school-based clinics do not provide counseling, referral or follow-up for family planning methods during the school year; nearly three-quarters do not provide prescriptions for contraceptives, and more than 80% avoid dispensing any contraceptives on site (Riessman, 1991). Thus there are a number of school-based health clinics which appear to successfully avoid these moral concerns.

Other researchers, however, assert that school-based facilities are inherently evil because they are inextricably tied to the promotion of abortion (Glasow, 1988). Richard Glasow, Education Director of the National Right to Life, points out that many school-based health clinics are supported (at least in part) by organizations that are not expressly anti-abortion and by some that promote pro-abortion policies and programs. He argues that because many school-based health clinics use Title X clinics as models for treating teens, they merely side-step the moral issue of abortion by establishing patterns of referrals to other clinics and other agencies that provide abortions and abortion counseling (Glasow, 1988).

Thus, some argue that a number of school-based health clinics were started and staffed by those who believe that artificial birth control and abortion are preferable to teenage pregnancy and parenting.[54] It is not

---

[53]   By 1991, the Center for Population Options reports that there were 306 school-based clinics in operation (Riessmann, 1991).

[54]   According to the Center for Population Options, however, this is a misrepresentation of their primary purpose. According to the Center for Population Options, the primary purpose of school-based and school-linked health clinics "is to provide young people, many of whom have no other regular source of medical care, with comprehensive health care" (Kirby, Waszak, & Ziegler, 1989: 11).

surprising that statements from church authorities are almost unanimous in their opposition to school-based health clinics "as they now exist" (Center for the Study of Family Development, 1991). The Florida Catholic Conference, for instance, *defines* school-based health clinics as health clinics on school property designed to provide birth control services to students (Florida Catholic Conference, 1986). Others reflecting this position include the Archdiocese of Boston, Bishop Leo T. Maher of San Diego, Archbishop Roger Mahony of Los Angeles, and Archbishop J. Francis Stafford of Denver (Archdiocese of Boston, 1986; Archdiocese of Denver, 1987; Maher, 1986).

On the other hand, Archbishop Pilarczyk writes that school-based health clinics could be "of considerable service" to youth if there were "ironclad reassurance that these clinics would not be or become, even in part, counseling agencies for contraceptives or for abortion" (1986). A close reading of the U.S. Bishops' *Statement on School-Based Clinics* (1987), also indicates the possibility that school-based clinics might be useful if they consistently avoid such moral quagmires. The Bishops of Connecticut and Archbishop Roach of the Archdiocese of Saint Paul and Minneapolis take similar positions (Roach, 1988; Connecticut Catholic Conference, 1987).

Health Education in Schools

Health education has been a part of many school curricula for decades. Health educators address a wide range of topics and issues from basic physiology and personal hygiene to more controversial topics such as sex education and life skill training. Some programs emphasize physiology; some emphasize the human reproductive system. In many curricula threats to the adolescents' health and well-being are addressed as separate units; avoidance of drug use and the effects of hallucinatory drugs and amphetamines might be studied in September, the need for good hygiene in October, and information about common venereal diseases in November. Often the only integrating factor in these topics is the impact on the biological person.

Among the primary topics covered in many programs is training for adolescents in the skills required to maintain healthy lifestyles. Such skills include responding to pressures to use drugs, alcohol, or tobacco or to engage in sexual activities. Additionally, research indicates that those adolescents who are more socially skilled in general, even apart from specific resistance skills, are more likely to be able to respond in a healthy manner to social pressure and are less likely to need the reinforcement offered by peers who engage in health-threatening behaviors (Elder & Stern, 1986). Programs incorporating such skill training, practice, and reinforcement have reported success, and have indicated that teens can learn to say no to early and nonmarital sex (Howard, 1985). Programs should also teach quite explicit communicative behaviors, should focus on interpersonal communication, problem-solving, and decision-making, and should emphasize consequences (Bonaguro, Rhonehouse, & Bonaguro, 1988; Elder & Stern, 1986).

Violence prevention has recently been added to the health curriculum of many schools. School-based violence programs often include topics such as conflict resolution, avoidance of handguns, peer mediation, the constructive channeling of anger, and dealing with aggression, bullying, and death (Wilson-Brewer, 1995).

Some topics are not presented for discussion because of the controversy they have previously engendered. Because of the belief that adolescents should not be sexually active, for example, some argue that promoting sexual responsibility is unnecessary or that it may encourage sexual experimentation (Blau & Gullotta, 1993). To the contrary, research indicates that, in general, exposure to sex education programs is related to knowledge about sexuality, conception, and contraception but not to sexual activity or pregnancy (Voydanoff & Donnelly, 1990). Because of the controversy surrounding sex education programs, many elementary and secondary schools do not offer any at all; many other curricula avoid emotionally heated topics such as homosexuality and masturbation (Orr, 1982; Blau & Gullotta, 1993). Avoidance of difficult topics by those with the responsibility to educate teens has not proven to be an effective deterrent to the many adolescents who become sexually active before reaching adulthood.

Perhaps as an outgrowth of the potential controversies involved in health education, many states do not require that health education be taught during middle or high school (Lovato, Allensworth, & Chan, 1989). Many professionals argue, however, that health education is very much needed as a separate and distinct subject within school curricula. They suggest that the primary goal of health education is "to provide students with the knowledge skills, and behaviors to choose a health-enhancing life-style" (Committee on School Health of the American Academy of Pediatrics, 1993: 105).

CHAPTER 6:

SUGGESTIONS FOR IMPROVING HEALTH CARE DELIVERY TO ADOLESCENTS

These issues, barriers, and problems with the existing adolescent health care system lead us to make a number of general suggestions toward its improvement and to present some program prototypes that address the challenges to adolescent health in a manner consistent with the precepts of Catholic moral teachings.

Five suggestions are presented here. First, it seems clear that the prevention of health problems among adolescents should be a central component of any health care system. Prevention and early intervention of adolescent health problems should address social morbidities as well as the biomedical and mental health problems of teenagers. Secondly, because so many adolescents engage in risky, health-compromising behaviors tied at least in part to their ignorance or rejection of fundamental life-affirming values, health care and health education should make an effort to articulate and promote such values to them. Health care and health education should be value-laden and, whenever possible, present to adolescents an ethical framework of life-affirming values consistent with those values articulated by Catholic moral theologians. The third suggestion for improving health care delivery to adolescents is that systems strive to be culturally competent and to recognize the diversity of cultures, ethnic heritages, and racial backgrounds of the teenagers in this country. The fourth suggestion is a call for the integration of service delivery. Fifth is to make every effort to encourage the appropriate use of health care services by adolescents and their families. Improvements along these lines would significantly improve the quality of health care for adolescents.

When possible, examples of programs addressing these suggestions are also presented. Since existing health-care programs and projects designed to deliver needed care to adolescents run the gamut from traditional doctors' offices to facilities with a full range of medical and social services, a broad range of programs is presented. Some are particularly successful at attracting patients from inner-city neighborhoods, some treat only a particular type of health condition, some are geared to attract all adolescents and steer them into more main-line facilities, while still others attempt to prevent the onset of social morbidities common to adolescence or a particular health-compromising behavior.

The existing projects also vary in their ability to affect the health and well-being of today's teens. Some projects have made remarkable strides in some areas but had no lasting effects in others. Evaluation of the worth of any particular approach entails an understanding that the goals of each project are different, the populations they hope to help are different, the assumptions and funding requirements of each are different and their outcomes are different as well. While no programs are perfect, some programs offer very helpful insights.

PREVENTION AND EARLY INTERVENTION

One way to reduce the difficulties associated with adolescent health problems is to prevent their onset. Clearly, reducing the number of cases of adolescents who contract an infectious disease or metabolic disorder is generally preferable to finding a "miracle" cure. Barring prevention, early intervention almost always makes treatment more effective. Both these approaches should be a primary focus for reducing the impact of the physical and mental conditions afflicting young people as well as those social morbidities disproportionately affecting their health. Medical practitioners, counselors, teachers, and parents would support the health and well-being of adolescents if preventive interventions were widely available to young people today.

Guidelines for Adolescent Preventive Services (GAPS)

Recently the American Medical Association published a full list of recommendations for primary care physicians caring for adolescent patients (Elster & Kuznets, 1994). Some of their recommendations reflect a national consensus of medical personnel; others were developed by a national scientific advisory board in response to their perceptions of adolescent health challenges in contemporary society. Their recommendations include preventive health guidance such as discussions with physicians on diet, fitness, adolescent development, and the avoidance of health-compromising behaviors such as smoking, sexual activity, and drug use. They include preventive screening for disorders such as tuberculosis, hypertension, and cervical cancer. In addition, the American Medical Association recommends a series of preventive inoculations and increased consultations with the adolescents' parents. Figure 6.1 presents a summary of the schedule of the preventive services they recommend for adolescents.

On the whole, these recommendations are remarkably consonant with those arising out of Catholic social teaching concerning adolescent health and health care. The recommendations are largely preventative and they acknowledge the complex nature of social morbidities. It is recommended, for example, that adolescents be questioned about tobacco, drugs and alcohol usage, experiences of physical and sexual abuse, and the existence of school problems, an eating disorder, or depression. Other recommendations include periodic screening for high blood pressure, elevated serum cholesterol levels, and STDs as well as consistent and repeated patient/physician discussions to promote and maintain healthy behaviors. As a reflection of the centrality of parents and families for healthy adolescent development, periodic parental contact with their teenager's physician is also recommended. The goal of these parental health guidance sessions would be to help parents adjust to the changing needs of their adolescents (Elster & Kuznets, 1994: 13).

The GAPS recommendations are not simply a codification of existent policies. They represent a shift in emphasis toward disease prevention and health promotion. Table 6.1 presents a summary of how the GAPS recommendations differ from the current system of health care delivery. The American Academy of Pediatrics developed a protocol entitled "The Injury Prevention Program" (TIPP) to help physicians work with patients towards a reduction in unintentional injuries. The "Put Prevention Into Practice" (PPIP) program, developed by the U.S. Public Health Service, provides medical staff information and tools for patient education and counseling including videos, posters, and warning stickers for patient files. Preventable problems such as tobacco use, lack of exercise, riding bicycles without helmets, early sexual activity, and access to firearms are targeted by this program (Paulson & Diguiseppi, 1995).

Prevention Projects

A few promising programs designed to address the problems of adolescence focus on the prevention of the behaviors and situations which are likely to eventually create a serious problem or crisis. These programs generally focus on providing adolescents with the resources they need to steer away

Figure 6.1: Recommended Frequency of Preventive Health Services by Age and Procedure

Procedure	Age of Adolescent		
	Early 11-14 years	Middle 15-17 years	Late 18-21 years
Health Guidance			
Parenting*	○	○	
Development	●	●	●
Diet and Fitness	●	●	●
Lifestyle**	●	●	●
Injury Prevention	●	●	●
Screening *History*			
Eating Disorders	●	●	●
Sexual Activity***	●	●	●
Alcohol and Other Drug Use	●	●	●
Tobacco Use	●	●	●
Abuse	●	●	●
School Performance	●	●	●
Depression	●	●	●
Risk for Suicide	●	●	●
Physical Assessment Blood Pressure	●	●	●
BMI	●	●	●
Comprehensive Exam	○	○	○

Procedure (cont.)	Early 11-14 years	Middle 15-17 years	Late 18-21 years
Tests			
Cholesterol	□-1	□-1	□-1
TB	□-2	□-2	□-2
GC, Clamydia, HPV	□-3	□-3	□-3
HIV, Syphilis	□-4	□-4	□-4
Pap Smear	□-5	□-5	●
Immunizations			
MMR	○		
Td		○	
HBV	□-6	□-6	□-6

● : Yearly
○: Once per time period
□: Yearly if in high risk category

* Parent health-guidance visit is recommended
** Includes counseling regarding sexual behavior and avoidance of tobacco, alcohol, and other drug use.
***Includes history of unintended pregnancy and STD

High Risk Categories:
1. Screening test perfomed if family history is positive for early cardiovascular diseas of hyperlipidemia.
2. Screen if positive for exposure to active TB or lives/works in high-risk situation
3. Screen if sexually active
4. Screen if high-risk for infection.
5. Screen annually if sexually active or 18 years or older.
6. Vaccinate if high-risk for hepatitis B infection

SOURCE: Elster & Kuznets, 1994, *AMA Guidelines for Adolescent Preventive Services (GAPS): Recommendations and Rationale:* Table 16.1:179.

TABLE 6.1: How GAPS Differs from the Traditional Practice of Medical Care for Adolescents

GAPS Recommendations	Traditional Medical Care
Preventive interventions provided by the physician complement health education that adolescents receive in their family, school, and community.	Physician role is generally considered independent of health education offered by family, schools, and the community.
Emphasis is on health promotion as well as disease prevention.	Diagnostic and therapeutic interventions are disease-oriented.
Preventive interventions target "social morbidities," such as alcohol and other drug use, suicide, STDs (including HIV), unintended pregnancy, and eating disorders.	Emphasis is on biomedical problems, including the medical consequences of health risk behaviors, such as STDs and pregnancy.
Emphasis is on screening for "co-morbidities," i.e., adolescent participation in clusters of specific health risk behaviors.	Emphasis is on the diagnosis and treatment of categorical health conditions.
Annual visits allow early detection of health problems and provide an opportunity for health guidance, immunizations, and the development of a therapeutic relationship.	Visits scheduled as needed for acute care episodes, follow-up care, management of chronic conditions, or sports examinations.
Comprehensive physical examinations are performed once during early, once during middle, and once during late adolescence.	Current standards vary from no recommendation on periodicity, to examinations every two years adolescence, to examinations required for participation in sports.
Parents receive health guidance at least twice during their child's adolescence.	The nature, type, and frequency of health guidance is left to the discretion of the physician.

SOURCE: Elster & Kuznets, 1994, *AMA Guidelines for Adolescent Preventive Services (GAPS): Recommendations and Rationale,* Table 1.2: xxv.

from health-compromising behaviors.

The goals of the projects presented here vary. The first focuses on healthy development by promoting adolescent well-being and preventing health-compromising behaviors. The others focus on more specific social morbidities such as the prevention of alcohol use, substance abuse, or violence by adolescents.

Promotion of Healthy Development

In anticipation of the many challenges adolescents face as they mature in American society, some programs attempt to provide them with added social and psychological resources before they meet with difficulties. Such primary prevention projects provide:

> . . . a set of strategies organized *before* a defined or unwanted situation or behavior occurs. Primary prevention is directed toward promoting well-being--a positive, healthy state. Primary prevention may mean inoculation against polio or measles, to give one example. This medical strategy requires people to present themselves for a shot. Quick, easy, and basically painless, this strategy does not place much responsibility on the individuals who deliver or receive the immunization. The inoculator must deliver good serum in the correct manner, and the population must show up. It is a relatively passive process, which requires minimal interaction. The effectiveness and ease of the "quick fix" method of prevention in the medical field may lead us to believe there can be a similar approach to problems of living.

> Primary prevention strategies are directed toward the underlying causes of such problems. Primary prevention involves enhancing the environments and building strengths in a general population . . . (Blumenkrantz, 1992: 28)

One such primary prevention strategy was created by David Blumenkrantz and is being used at a number of sites throughout the United States. The *Rite of Passage Experience* is a collaborative effort which involves the young people, their parents, their schools, and the social services agencies in their communities. It provides for the adolescents a ceremonial ritual of initiation into adulthood, provides structured challenges to young people and their families, and teaches young people the knowledge and skills that are essential for them to become happy and healthy adults. This program is designed "to promote good physical health and nutrition, develop decision-making and problem-solving skills, build competencies, increase self-esteem, and most important, enhance the support systems that help strengthen links among and between schools, family, community, and peers" (Blumenkrantz, 1992:41).

Evaluations of the teens who were provided with this *Rite of Passage Experience* during the sixth grade indicate that they are significantly more involved with their families, have more positive attitudes toward school, have engaged in fewer delinquent acts, are less alienated, and have lower rates of drugs and alcohol use (Blumenkrantz, 1992). These differences appear to hold up over at least a few years.

Prevention of Alcohol Use, Substance Abuse, and Violence

Some preventive projects are a bit more focused; they seek to change more limited patterns of behavior. For instance, some such promising programs concentrate on the prevention of alcohol consumption by adolescents. Some programs are focused on the provision of information concerning the dangers of alcohol consumption, some seek to alter the adolescents' goal setting abilities and decisionmaking skills, others try to develop the young person's ability to resist social pressures (Hansen, 1993). Research results indicate that programs which change the normative beliefs of teenagers concerning the acceptability and prevalence of alcohol consumption among their peers are among the more effective programs (Hansen, 1993). Programs which are initiated *before* teens establish patterns of alcohol consumption are more effective than those which seek to intervene once the underage drinking has become frequent.

A community-based program for the prevention of substance abuse instituted in Kansas City during the mid-1980's also shows promise. This substance abuse program was directed at sixth and seventh grade students; its goals included the prevention of use of tobacco, marijuana, and alcohol among young teens. This program sought to prevent drug abuse among adolescents by a school-based educational program emphasizing skills needed to resist peer-pressure, mass-media programming, parent education programs, peer-leader intervention, and the involvement of community organizations. The analysis of self-reported data indicates that significantly fewer teens involved in the program than in other similar areas initiated the use of these substances for at least a year after the start of the program (Pentz, Dwyer, MacKinnon, Flay, Hansen, Wang, & Johnson, 1989; Vincent, Clearie, & Schluchter, 1987).

Two other substance abuse programs with positive results are *Project ALERT* and *Project SHOUT*. Both focused on the prevention of tobacco use by young people in junior high schools, but *Project ALERT* also included efforts to reduce the use of marijuana among these students.

Project SHOUT, which involved nearly 3000 teens in the San Diego area, had an emphasis on interpersonal behavior aimed at countering peer pressure to initiate smoking and the use of chewing tobacco. A unique feature of the program was the use of telephone and mail contact with the participants to reinforce the messages taught in the classroom. The evaluation of this program indicates that it is a cost-effective intervention which appears to significantly alter the tobacco usage of teens for at least the first three years after their exposure to the program (Elder, Wildey, de Moor, Sallis, Eckhardt, Edwards, Erickson, Golbbeck, Hovell, Johnston, Levitz, Molgaard, Young, Vito, & Woodruff, 1993).

Similarly, the results from *Project ALERT* indicate that this social-influence model of intervention was relatively successful in preventing the initiation of smoking and marijuana use among participants. The curriculum presented through this program helps students to develop reasons not to use these drugs, "identify pressures to use them, counter pro-drug messages, learn how to say no to external and internal pressures, understand that most people do not use drugs, and recognize the benefits of resistance" (Ellickson & Bell, 1990: 1300).

Over the past few years a number of prevention and intervention programs have been designed to reduce youth violence (Wilson-Brewer, 1995). In addition to those developed through the Centers for Disease Control and Prevention, more than 800 prevention strategies have been developed by organizations such as the Interagency Task Force on Violence Prevntion, the Carnegie Corporation, the National Crime Prevention Council, Education Development Center, the Children's Defense Fund, and the Center for the Study and Prevention of Violence (Wilson-Brewer, 1995). Some are school-based, some emphasize community linkages, and still others stem from health clinics. The effects of these programs are, however, as yet largely undocumented (Tolan, & Guerra, 1994).

Prevention Programs for Pregnant or Parenting Adolescents

Some successful programs are directed toward those adolescents who have previously engaged in a specific health-compromising behavior. These programs are designed to alleviate some of the negative health and social consequences of those behaviors and prevent the teen from repeating them in the future. For instance, a number of programs were funded by the Federal Government in response to the programming needs of parenting and pregnant adolescents who bring their pregnancies to term.[55]

---

[55] The original Adolescent Family Life Act, Title XX of the Public Health Service Act, was passed in 1981 and funding has continued at least through 1995 (Office of Adolescent Pregnancy Programs, 1990). Through the Office

One of the more successful projects developed and distributed a value-based curriculum for pregnant adolescents and their families. This program--*A Community of Caring*--recognizes the importance of ethical and family values immediately necessary for these adolescents.[56]   It is comprised of teaching modules which are designed "to help the adolescent mothers, fathers, and their families understand how to have a healthy pregnancy, a safe delivery, and give their infants a good start in life" (Joseph P. Kennedy, Jr. Foundation, 1982: 1). Some of the modules focus on the physical facts about pregnancy and childbirth. Many, however, deal with developing the skills needed for the teens to make pro-social and healthy decisions in the future. This curriculum seeks to teach virtues such as love, trust, patience, commitment, courage, loyalty and compassion. It also seeks to demonstrate to the young participants the impact of their decisions on their child's quality of life, their own life chances, and those of the people they love (Joseph P. Kennedy, Jr. Foundation, 1982). Evaluation results indicate positive outcomes in some instances, ambiguous outcomes in others (Miller & Dyk, 1991).

Among the other encouraging projects funded through the Adolescent Family Life Act and directed at pregnant and parenting teens and their families, was one which stressed the importance of logical and systematic decision-making. This project entailed a counseling approach rather than an educational approach. A central tenet of the *Chance to Grow* project concerns the importance of the adolescent's parenting decision. Therefore, releasing for adoption was presented to the participants as a positive option within the structured decision-making counseling program (Office of Adolescent Pregnancy Programs, 1990). Over the course of its funding, this project was able to demonstrate a postponement in repeat sexual activity by the participants, an increased likelihood that these adolescents would

---

of Adolescent Pregnancy Programs, Office of Population Affairs, Department of Health and Human Services, it has provided funding for organizations to help find effective strategies for service provision to pregnant adolescents, adolescent parents, and their families. The funded projects are required to offer a broad range of services to the teens including primary health care services, maternity and adoption counseling, educational services relating to family life and problems relating to premarital sexual relations (*Federal Register*, 1989: 52909).

[56]   This project was developed under the auspices of the Joseph P. Kennedy, Jr. Foundation. Further funding of the curriculum and its associated manuals, teachers' guide, and handouts was received from the Office of Adolescent Pregnancy Programs (Joseph P. Kennedy, Jr. Foundation, 1982; Office of Adolescent Pregnancy Programs, 1990).

release their children for adoption, as well as some socio-economic benefits of participation to the young mother (Donnelly, 1992; Donnelly & Davis-Berman, 1994).

The teaching of chastity:

San Diego, Jan 14-- Lori Brown, 14, is practicing how to say no to sex, learning strategies to save her virginity.

Her instructor is Dajahn Blevins, a health educator from the Urban League here, who plays the role of the girl's would-be seducer and tests her with the crude patois of the street and the sweet promises of a fairy tale.

Mr. Blevins tells Lori that she is the only girl at Roosevelt Junior High School who is not "hooking up." He says it's time to "take your panties off" or be dumped for someone who will.

She looks him straight in the eye and says, "No," just as she was taught, without excuse or explanation.

Still, he badgers her saying she must be stuck up or scared. The he whispers that he wants her so badly he will do anything: beg, crawl, buy her expensive gifts.

But Lori is stteadfast. "Stop pressuring me," she says, "I'm not into that now. I'm into education."

SOURCE: Gross, 1994, Copyright ©1994 The New York Times. Reprinted by Permission.

VALUE-LADEN HEALTH CARE AND HEALTH EDUCATION

Adolescents, as they strive to become autonomous, are faced with decision after decision with the potential to enhance or damage their health and well-being. Since most of these decisions hinge largely on the moral dimension, their families, health care providers, and educators are challenged to provide them with an ethical framework which will form the foundation for appropriate decisions. This framework necessarily involves a number of underlying values or assumptions concerning such basic understandings as the nature of human development and the value of human life. Those frameworks which are both internally consistent and explicit will provide the most useful foundation for decision-making.

For some of the players involved in the support of adolescent well-being, the adoption or promotion of internally consistent and explicit values presents a demanding challenge. The parents of adolescents generally have the best opportunity to impart the values to their children unimpeded by legal or organizational considerations. It is within families that children are expected to first develop their moral characters. It is within families that there is continued access to the intensity of relationship upon which most learning is contingent. As the inventory of social morbidities common among adolescents illustrates, however, some families have thus far been unable to meet the challenge of providing teenagers with an ethical framework of life-affirming values which allow adolescents to consistently protect their own health and well-being.

Therefore, other groups and institutions are being challenged to provide clear and uncompromising standards and values to adolescents as they make important decisions concerning health-compromising behaviors (Hansen, 1993; Prager, 1993; Ryan, 1993).

Teaching Values and Morality in the Schools

Some schools are refocusing efforts to present ethical standards and moral systems to their students (Lickona, 1993a). Many educators have come to recognize that many children are no longer learning the values needed for productive community participation in their homes. These educators have come to the common realization:

> . . .that we do share a basic morality, essential for our survival; that adults must promote this morality by teaching the young, directly and indirectly, such values as respect, responsibility, trustworthiness, fairness, caring, and civic virtue; and that these values are not merely subjective preferences but that they have objective worth and a claim on our collective conscience.

> Such values affirm our human dignity, promote the good of the individual and the common good, and protect our human rights.

> They define our responsibilities in a democracy, and they are recognized by all civilized people and taught by all enlightened creeds. *NOT* to teach children these core ethical values is a grave moral failure. (emphasis in the original {Lickona, 1993a: 9})

For schools and the other groups involved in the health and well-being of adolescents, the task to present fundamental values is significantly more complex than it is for families (Berreth & Scherer, 1993). In the United States, publicly-funded institutions must rely on values which are common throughout the diverse ethnic and religious communities they serve. Schools, for example, might promote curricula which teach those values espoused in the Constitution and the Bill of Rights or they might rely on students to discuss ethical dilemmas. Adolescents who understand that their decisions have a moral component, that they are members of a community and individuals with rights and responsibilities, should be better prepared for sound (and healthy) decision-making.

Some educators argue that the moral dimension of adolescents' development should go beyond such secular values and include more religiously-based systems in their curricula. This presents a challenge in a pluralist society that mandates the separation of Church and State. One approach to the problem of teaching values in public institutions is to present explicitly "Christian," "Muslim," and "Jewish" teachings as well as more secular ethical frameworks to the students, allowing the students to choose among them.

This approach (and its more secular versions) is generally called the values clarification approach. Some versions of this approach have been used in connection with a number of health-impacting decisions. Its detractors point out that often the teachers fail to distinguish between personal preferences and moral values (Lickona, 1993a).

Partially in response to allegations that it is not enough to present various value systems to young people, educators have developed another approach. The character education model is designed to promote *particular* values to the students in an attempt to lead them to more responsible behaviors. In public schools and institutions these values are often secular ones such as "honesty" and "fairness" which are acceptable to almost all segments of the community (Huffman, 1993). Some character education programs make a concerted effort to select the value traits to be promoted in the public schools through consultation with parents and other community members. One school district involved in the *Personal Responsibility Education Process (PREP)* program, for example, selected a number of values including "compassion," "assertiveness," "discretion," and "respect" through the consensus of a community-based committee (Moody & McKay, 1993).

Private schools and organizations, however, are afforded an opportunity to embrace, articulate, and support the value system they find most cogent even if it involves some religiously-based components. Some private schools, precisely because they are *not* confronted with legal requirements to present a range of ethical frameworks or a so-called "value-free" approach, choose to present a single, and perhaps more fully articulated, ethical framework in their curricula. This tactic can be seen as a religion-based version of the character education approach. In some schools, the ethical framework is openly labeled "Biblical," in some "Roman Catholic," and in others "Jewish" or "Muslim."

It is important to note that while the articulation of appropriate moral and ethical frameworks for decision-making appears to be a necessary component of health education, there is little evidence to believe that any school program is sufficient "cure" to the health-threatening decisions among teenagers. Neither the values clarification approach to moral education nor the character education approach has been shown to be a great direct influence over adolescents' behaviors (Leming, 1993; Lockwood, 1993). There is, in fact, a paucity of evidence to suggest that young peoples' behaviors are a direct result of the values they are taught in most existing programs.

Nevertheless, because so many of the health issues facing adolescents, their families, and health care providers are inextricably tied to important moral or ethical questions, health care policies, programs, organizations, and decisions have a responsibility to provide the clearest moral foundation possible. An emphasis on the value of all human life, for instance, is a relatively unambiguous moral precept of Catholic theology and broader Christian teaching. The application of this precept would have far-reaching consequences even if only consistently applied by young people of faith. These adolescents, when confronted by decisions regarding violence, suicide, reckless driving, drug use, or abortion would make their decisions concerning these health-compromising behaviors informed by a clearer understanding of their own moral foundation.

Educating for Abstinence and Sexual Responsibility

One of the central tenets of Christian teaching which would, if taken seriously, make a crucial impact on the health-compromising behaviors of adolescents, is the belief that "sexual intercourse is best in the context of lifelong marriage" (Reiss, 1994). Most sex education programs for adolescents[57] that have been presented to teens in this country, however, do not emphasize the value of nonmarital sexual abstinence[58]. There have been

---

[57]   There are fewer programs still emphasizing chastity for unmarried persons of all ages.

[58]   Some writers prefer the term "chastity" over "sexual abstinence" because it is not applicable to the avoidance of other activities such as drinking alcohol or eating desserts. However, since most of the academic and professional literature uses "abstinence" when referring to programs designed to reduce

a wide variety of emphases in the sex education programs offered in recent years. Some focus on reproduction while others include information about contraception, sexually transmitted diseases, values clarification, peer relationships, sexual responsibility, and communication and decision-making skills (Voydanoff & Donnelly, 1990).

There are a number of reasons why, despite their prevalence, there has been little reduction in early sexual activity attributable to prevention programs. Often they are brief and superficial; programs that are superficial consistently can be shown to have little or no impact on the participants. Furthermore, most of the educational programs take place in junior and senior high schools after a substantial minority of the students have already become sexually active (Blau & Gullotta, 1993; Voydanoff & Donnelly, 1990).

Another important factor is that most pregnancy prevention and abstinence programs are aimed exclusively at adolescents. Doing so ignores both the importance of modeling behaviors and the prevalence of adult/teen sexual contact (Males, 1993a). More specifically, focusing exclusively on teenagers overlooks the strong relationship between adult and adolescent behaviors. Males (1993a: 431) cites very strong correlations, for example, between the annual rates of births, unwed births, STDs and abortions for teens and adults.[59] In a very real sense most of the prevention projects call for adolescents to behave *more responsibly* than the many adults in the society.

A second and crucial factor is that most sexual contact is between pairs with a significant age discrepancy. The children of most teen mothers are fathered by adults (Males, 1993a):

> Even if every U.S. high school male abstained from intercourse or used a condom perfectly, 75% to 80% of all births and a similar percentage of STDs among teen-age females still would occur. (Males, 1993: 432)

If this age pattern was taken seriously, programs would include males in their twenties who have long-since left high school.

Since the early 1980's a number of programs have been designed to

---

nonmarital adolescent sexual activity, it is the term more frequently used in this document.

[59] The correlations cited by Males have statistically significant Pearson r product-moment coefficent values of .934 (all births), .919 (unwed births), .884 (abortion rates), and .966 (STD rates). Birth and unwed birth rates were calculated annually from 1940 to 1990, abortion rates from 1973-1988, and STD rates from 1956-1990 (Males, 1993a: 431).

promote abstinence among adolescents by presenting it as the most effective method of avoiding the health risks associated with early sexual activity and pregnancy. Many of these programs have been labeled "abstinence-only" programs because they have been funded through private and Federal grants that proscribe the distribution of information concerning artificial means of birth control, access to such contraceptive devices, and information about or referrals for abortions. Most were developed in reaction to sex education programs that included information concerning contraception and techniques of avoiding sexually transmitted diseases:

> Concerned that sex education programs were "value-free," developers of these programs consistently emphasized the message that youth should not engage in intercourse until marriage. To avoid sending a "double-message," programs discussed abstinence only and did not discuss contraception. (Kirby, 1992:281)

Such programs are often politically palatable in arenas where other programs would face resistance on the part of some parents or other vocal segments of the community (Jorgensen, Potts, & Camp, 1993; Lickona, 1993b).

A number of the abstinence programs which do not cover any information about contraception have gained a good deal of notoriety. *Project Taking Charge*, for example, is an abstinence-based intervention for seventh-grade students that was first offered in Wilmington, Delaware, Ironton, Ohio, and West Point, Mississippi (Jorgensen, 1991; Jorgensen, Potts, & Camp, 1993). In addition to information concerning the importance of abstaining from nonmarital sexual activity, this project includes instructional units covering self-development, anatomy, physiology, sexually transmitted diseases, vocational goal setting, family values, and communication. Evaluation results indicate that participants and their parents demonstrated increased levels of knowledge concerning anatomy, physiology, complications caused by adolescent pregnancy, and sexually transmitted diseases (Jorgensen, Potts, & Camp, 1993). Furthermore these cognitive gains lasted for at least the first six months following completion of the program. Data from the six-month followup study also indicate that this program may have helped the participants to delay initiation of sexual activity (Jorgensen, Potts, & Camp, 1993).

Other influential, abstinence-focused programs which do not cover any information about contraception include the *Sex Respect* and *Sexuality, Commitment and Family: Me, My World, My Future* curricula. These programs are being used in a number of sites throughout the country (Howard, 1992; Department of Health and Human Services, Office of Population Affairs, Office of Adolescent Pregnancy Programs, 1990;

Lickona, 1993b). Evaluation results in terms of their ability to postpone or reduce sexual activity among teens are unclear.[60] Unfortunately, use of the *Sex Respect* curriculum in public schools has been labeled "controversial" in some areas and has come under legal scrutiny in others (Granberry, 1994; Tuck, 1991; Times-Picayune, Nov. 23, 1991, p.3). The values espoused through this program are so representative of conservative Christian teachings that constitutional questions of separation of Church and State have been raised in a Louisiana case (Ponessa, 1993; Roman, 1993).

At least one abstinence-focused intervention appears to delay the start of intercourse among adolescents. This program--*Postponing Sexual Involvement*--was funded by the Department of Health and has been used in the Atlanta area (Howard, 1992; Department of Health and Human Services, Office of Population Affairs, Office of Adolescent Pregnancy Programs, 1990). This program, however, is based on aspects of social learning theory which suggest that young people will be able to resist social pressure to engage in health compromising behaviors such as sexual activity if they are taught the tools and techniques necessary for risk avoidance (Bandura, 1986; Kirby, 1992; Kirby, 1993; Howard, 1992).

One of the best known abstinence interventions in the nation, this program involves classroom instruction and peer counseling. The classroom sessions are presented to eighth graders and involve presentation of techniques and tools to help them postpone sexual activity, as well as basic human sexuality information including contraceptive information. The peer counselors are trained eleventh and twelfth-grade students. A longitudinal, five year evaluation indicates that students experiencing this program were much more likely to delay initiating sexual activity during their high school years (Howard, 1992).

The sum total of the evaluation results of abstinence-focused programs, however, is not entirely clear. The evaluations of many are clouded because sexual activity is not a clearly designated outcome variable (Adamek & Thoms, 1991; Kirby, 1993; Olsen, Weed, Nielsen, & Jensen, 1992; Roosa & Christopher, 1990). Some studies focus, for example, on changes in attitudes or knowledge or pregnancy rates--none of which correspond directly to sexual activity. From the perspective of the educator, this oversight is understandable:

> Few other classes or programs are evaluated by observing change exhibited outside-school. The effectiveness of English classes is not evaluated by measuring improvement in the English spoken off campus,

---

[60] Evaluation results do indicate that teens exposed to this program found it somewhat helpful and that the younger participants evaluated it more positively than the older ones (Olsen, Weed, Nielsen, & Jensen, 1992).

and the effectiveness of civic classes is not assessed by measuring the law-abiding behavior of students. (Kirby, 1992: 280)

Thus, an expectation that reductions in sexual activity will result from the participation in a particular school-based program requires evaluation "criteria which are far more demanding, and perhaps unrealistic, than are criteria for the effectiveness of other school programs" (Kirby, 1992).

In most cases where actual sexual activity has been measured, no significant changes can be documented (Christopher & Roosa, 1990; Kirby, 1993; Roosa & Christopher, 1990). With only a few exceptions, evaluation results of the effectiveness of abstinence-only programs in terms of their actual ability to alter the behavior of teens are not particularly encouraging (Christopher & Roosa, 1990; Hayes, 1987; Moore & Wertheimer, 1984; Roosa & Christopher, 1990; Roosa & Christopher, 1992; Thiel & McBride, 1992; Voydanoff & Donnelly, 1990).

Detractors of abstinence-only programs point out that many of the curricula are fear-based; many curricula present all of the dangers of nonmarital intercourse without making a realistic appraisal of the immense social pressures that foster early sexual activity (Brick & Roffman, 1993; Lickona, 1993b). Educators have demonstrated that positive language--in this case emphasizing that postponement of sexual activity until marriage is a positive health decision--is likely to be a far more effective mechanism than is a fear-based approach (Brooks & Kann, 1993).

A few positive results can, however, be cited. Educational programs that promote abstinence appear to be most effective when they are part of an overall preventive strategy which is directed toward the elementary school-age adolescent. Very young adolescents and pre-pubertal adolescents, it appears, are better able than older adolescents to benefit from programs which emphasize abstinence (Barth, Leland, Kirby, & Fetro, 1992; Haynes, 1993; Howard, 1992; Howard & McCabe, 1992; Miller, Norton, Jensen, Lee, Christopherson, & King, 1993; Nicholson & Postrado, 1992). In their evaluation of three different abstinence-focused programs, Olsen, Weed, Neilsen, and Jensen (1992) concluded that junior-high school aged female students and those who have remained chaste[61] and uninformed of birth control information are the ones who consistently rate these programs most positively.

---

[61] The term used by these authors was "virgin-naive" rather than uninformed and chaste. The respondents were classified according to their previous sexual behavior and their previous knowledge of contraceptive information into three categories: "nonvirgin," "virgin-informed," and "virgin-naive." The programs examined were *Values and Choices, Teen Aid,* and *Sex Respect* (Olsen, Weed, Neilson, & Jensen, 1992).

Abstinence as a component of a more comprehensive preventive program appears to have a greater chance of affecting the behaviors of adolescents. As much research has pointed out, effective programs are comprehensive and intensive. Effective programs are more likely than ineffective ones to meet with the participants often, over a long period of time, and to be run by people perceived to be intensively involved with the young people (Miller, Card, Paikoff, & Peterson, 1992; Voydanoff & Donnelly, 1990). Superficial contact with a teacher or counselor or physician is unlikely to alter behaviors that are defined as acceptable, desirable, expected, and moral by large and powerful members of society. Programs that have been effective in delaying the start of sexual activity "generally include some combination of values and knowledge-based education, decision making and social skills training, reproductive health services, and alternatives or options that enhance motivation to avoid adolescent pregnancy" (Miller, Card, Paikoff, & Peterson, 1992: 271). They rely on curricula which allow the student to personalize the skills and information in ways necessary for successful avoidance of early sexual activity (Kirby, 1992).

CULTURALLY COMPETENT HEALTH CARE SERVICES

Health care professionals will be more effective if they take into account their own cultural biases and the cultural diversity of their clients. Health care providers have a culture which is very different from that of adolescents and most of their families. While studying to become physicians, nurses, and counselors, for example, the health care providers learn the "scientific" names and explanations for maladies and their cures. They are presented with vast information concerning technological and pharmaceutical responses to illness and they are taught which conditions warrant responses and which are ignorable. As Press points out:

> . . .biomedical jargon is designed to allow standardized teaching of medicine and standardized communication between medical professionals. It is *not* designed for physician-patient interaction. It serves the physician's ends--not the patient's, and reflects special training, not powers. (emphasis in the original {Press, 1982: 191})

Even well-educated adults who have not studied medicine or its allied fields often have difficulty comprehending medical jargon; it is all the more difficult for the young person with an often more limited understanding of biomedical terminology to understand information they may receive from their physician. Practitioners who realize that they are members of a distinct subculture because of their training and education will also understand that they must translate their explanations and instructions into terms which are more meaningful to their patients.

Furthermore, because adolescents in this country are culturally diverse, health care systems should be designed to be as "culturally competent" as possible. The culturally competent health care system is one which values cultural diversity, recognizes the dynamics involved when cultures interact, and can work effectively with the strengths of each individual cultural system (Cross, Bazran, Dennis, & Isaacs, 1989; U.S. Congress, Office of Technology Assessment, 1991c). Such a health care system would be staffed with individuals who are aware of their own cultural biases and "who are sensitive to cultural differences within as well as across racial and ethnic groups" (U.S. Congress, Office of Technology Assessment, 1991c: 190). A culturally competent health care system for adolescents would also include a more proportionate representation of minority practitioners. While not guaranteed to reduce the impact of inherent bias, racism, or lack of understanding, increasing the proportion of minority doctors, nurses, and other staff would be a reasonable goal.

INTEGRATED, COMMUNITY-BASED
SERVICE DELIVERY

Integrated services are oriented to treating the whole person in the context of the community in which they live and develop. Whole person in this context includes the physical, mental, and moral dimensions referred to in Chapter Three. Integrated health care also is designed to address the broad range of developmental and biopsychosocial needs of adolescents as well as the clustering of problems within individuals and families.

Based on an analysis of the evaluations of 13 different sorts of integrated health care programs, Schorr and Both (1991) conclude that successful programs have a number of common attributes. They are comprehensive, flexible, and responsive and deal with the child as an individual and as part of a family, and with the family as part of a neighborhood and a community. Staff in successful programs have the time, training, skills, and institutional support necessary to create an accepting environment and to build relationships of trust and respect with children and families. Furthermore, successful programs are well managed, usually by highly competent, energetic, committed and responsible individuals with clearly identifiable skills and attitudes. These include a willingness to experiment and take risks, tolerate ambiguity, work with diverse constituencies, and operate with a collaborative management style.

Successful programs are based on a client-centered and preventive orientation (Schorr & Both, 1991).

As mentioned earlier, the fragmentation of services is an important barrier to the delivery of adolescent health care. Several integrated approaches to health care delivery attempt to overcome these barriers. In order to balance the need for parental participation and the distinctive characteristics of the adolescent population, the most promising approach appears to be community-based adolescent health centers that provide a wide range of services to treat diverse problems including biomedical health problems, mental health problems, and social morbidities.

Integrated, community-based adolescent health care centers offer the possibility of programs easily accessed by adolescents, programs that also foster the involvement of families, and allow a full range of community groups and organizations to have input into the health care of young people. Some community-based facilities are closely tied to established medical facilities such as hospitals or public clinics, others are outgrowths of social service agencies. *Teen-Link* in Durham, North Carolina, for example, serves adolescents who are economically disadvantaged and previously under-served. Its program goals include the provision of "knowledge, skills, and alternative sources of social and medical support necessary to develop positive attitudes and behavior" among teens aged 10 to 18 (DuRant, 1991:450). This award-winning health program involves the county health and social service departments, local churches, public and private school systems, Duke University Medical Center, a family-oriented medical center, civic organizations, businesses, and the public housing authority (DuRant, 1991; Lincoln Community Health Center Brochure and private communication, 1993).

A full range of services is provided by the staff of this facility. Services include a number of primary-prevention programs to promote healthy behaviors, dental health care, comprehensive primary health care, prenatal services, nutritional counseling, other specialty medical services, WIC services, and mental health services (DuRant, 1991; Lincoln Community Health Center Brochure and private communication, 1993). These services are offered on-site or in some cases in the homes of the young people:

> Services are provided by a team of multidisciplinary professionals with special training in adolescent health issues. In addition to the health care providers, the staff includes outreach workers to conduct home visits and follow-up and a community health facilitator who lives in the community and recruits adolescents to the program through personal contact with the adolescents and their families. The health care team also includes a nutritionist who provides exercise programs and diet counseling for the adolescent patient. (DuRant, 1991:450-451)

Another equally innovative community-based health project for adolescents is *The Bridge Over Troubled Water* project in Boston. This project serves runaway youth in Boston who are between the ages of 12 and 21 and aims to help them leave the street. Unlike *Teen-Link*, however, the services are provided in a mobile medical van which moves around the city, improving access to its services. *The Bridge* offers health and social services such as drug and alcohol abuse counseling, dental care, acute medical care, vocational education, laboratory screening for sexually transmitted diseases and other infectious diseases including hepatitis, pregnancy testing, and prenatal and contraceptive counseling. The staff of this project are also multi-disciplinary and have been very successful in reaching a very high-risk population of adolescents (DuRant, 1991: 451).

FAMILY-CENTERED ADOLESCENT HEALTH CARE

The earlier discussion of Catholic moral and social teachings also emphasizes the importance of a family perspective in the development of adolescent health care policies and programs. Catholic teaching stresses the family as the foundation of the church, the society, and the community. A family perspective involves viewing individuals in the context of their family relationships and using the quality of family relationships as a criterion to assess the impact of policies and programs (Lynch & Preister, 1988). Policies and programs derived from a family perspective support and supplement family functioning, encourage and reinforce family commitment and stability, recognize the strength of family ties even when they are problematic, consider families as partners in service delivery, recognize the diversity of family life, and target vulnerable families (Consortium of Family Organizations, 1990; Ooms, 1990). A family perspective provides a framework for policy that addresses the broader context in which family-related problems occur.

This context can be understood by viewing human development as occurring in relation to four societal levels, each nested within the next according to its immediacy to the developing person. The most immediate level consists of a network of face-to-face relationships experienced by an individual including family, peer, and school-based relationships. The second level is the interlinked system of personal relationships in which an individual participates, such as linkages between the family and the school. The third level includes the external environments in which a person does not participate but which exert indirect influences, such as the work settings of family members. Finally, the broadest level consists of the belief systems and institutional patterns that provide the context for human development.[62]

This model provides a framework for looking at the ways in which families are interdependent with other aspects of society. For example, Chapter Two documented the importance of the media (a component of the broad cultural system) for adolescent health. Earlier chapters also show the profound impact of poverty derived from difficulties on the exosystem level on the health problems and care of adolescents. This approach makes clear that policies based on a family perspective also must be assessed in the context of other institutions such as the economy, community organizations, and government.

This family perspective is consistent with Catholic teaching on subsidiarity which recognizes the importance of addressing problems on the appropriate societal level and with communitarianism which posits that individuals, families and local communities such as neighborhoods exist prior to more institutionalized levels (see Chapter Three). Teachings on the preferential option for the poor acknowledge the difficulties that people as individuals have in addressing the broader social forces that create and maintain poverty on a societal level.

Furthermore, a good deal of more secular research suggests that adolescent health care should be family-centered. Family-centered health care treats the entire family, rather than just the teenager, as the focus of concern. Successful attempts at family-focused treatment of adolescents are cognizant of the impact that the policies and procedures, staffing, training, financing, recordkeeping, and the structure and organization of the program or agency itself have on the families involved (Snyder & Ooms, 1992).

Family-focused programs for adolescents frequently center on the treatment of social morbidities. Drug and alcohol abuse, violence and other forms of delinquency, mental health problems, adolescent pregnancy, and obesity and eating disorders are morbidities which are often treated through family-centered care (Miller, Card, Paikoff, & Peterson, 1992; Snyder & Ooms, 1992). Results of some studies, for example, indicate that open communication between parents and adolescents is associated with abstinence (Olson, Wallace, & Miller, 1984; Pick de Weiss, Atkin, Gribble, & Andrade-Palos, 1991). While few families do talk openly about sex, programs directed toward parents can increase the likelihood of this occurring (Howard, 1985; Warren & Neer, 1986). This research provides a strong rationale for providing parallel programs for parents and teens (Brown & Fritz, 1988).

The range of services offered by some of the successful programs is quite broad. Some are privately funded while others have been developed

---

[62] These levels are referred to by Bronfenbrenner (1986) as the microsystem, the mesosystem, the exosystem, and the macrosystem respectively.

by public agencies. The state of Delaware, for example, consolidated most children's and adolescent services into one unified department called "Department of Services for Children, Youth, and Their Families" (McCarthy, 1992). Subsumed into this agency were protective services, mental health services, alcohol and drug abuse treatment, and youth rehabilitative services. All staff receive intensive pro-family training to facilitate the use of family-focused interventions and the agency reviews all policies, procedures and laws in an attempt to maintain an organization which is responsive to the needs of each of the families it encounters (McCarthy, 1992). The range of services offered by another successful program in Montgomery County, Maryland, is somewhat narrower. This agency focuses primarily on the treatment of adolescent mental health and addiction problems. A previously existing family crisis intervention program called *Parents and Children Together (PACT)* was restructured in the late 1980's as a single point of entry for all families with adolescents experiencing substance abuse difficulties. *PACT* practitioners provide assessment and case management services to the families and adolescents, referral to appropriate community-based agencies, and continued involvement throughout the treatment (Luongo, 1992). Such programs have been successful not only in improving the chances for altered behaviors on the part of the adolescents and families involved, but they have also proved effective in reducing duplication of services, both the human and financial costs of out-of-home placements, and the appropriate distribution of treatment to those in need.

ENCOURAGING AGE-APPROPRIATE USE OF HEALTH CARE SERVICES

The final suggestion for improving the health care services of adolescents involves making existing services more accessible to adolescents and their families and more attuned to their developmental needs. Health promotion and health care presume that the patient recognizes that help is needed. Such help--which might consist of either changes in attitudes, knowledge and behaviors or changes in medical interventions--must then also be accessible to the adolescent. An increase in the health-related knowledge of adolescents and changes in patterns of their health-compromising behaviors necessitate a broad change in their social world. One potential avenue to such changes is through the mass media. Once adolescents and their parents have identified their need for medical intervention, those services must be available and accessible to this distinctive population. Those who provide health care services to teenagers, furthermore, should be cognizant of their unique developmental attributes.

Using the Mass Media for Health Promotion

The mass media have the potential to increase health-related knowledge and positively influence the decisions and behaviors of adolescents. People are exposed to information about health and illness throughout the print media, radio, movies, and on TV. For most Americans, the form of media with the greatest potential for influence is probably television. Many people indicate that television is their primary source of information about certain diseases such as cancer or AIDS (Freimuth, Stein, & Kean, 1989; Signorielli, 1993; Wallack, 1990).

Such information can be transferred to audiences within the context of programs, through public service announcements, or through news programs. Often program episodes focus on a particular health issue; programs which present these issues and their remedies somewhat realistically help to increase the viewer's health-related knowledge[63] (Montgomery, 1990; Signorielli, 1993). Program episodes with proactive health messages have aired on such topics as underage consumption of alcohol, smoking, AIDS, and drug abuse. While it is clear that entertainment television in a few instances has made a contribution to the public health awareness, it has very often also promoted unhealthy behaviors:

> The pro-social scenes and dialogue in the programs are often in conflict with the carefully crafted commercials that punctuate the programming with increasing frequency. So, while characters in popular sitcoms warn each other, from time to time, about the dangers of drinking, slick ads in other parts of the schedule repeatedly drive home the message that beer and wine are essential to the good life. (Montgomery, 1990: 127)

A second potential source of health-impacting messages is found within health-promoting campaigns. For example, recent health promotion TV campaigns have been used to spread information concerning the dangers of cigarette smoking, drug use, alcohol consumption, and AIDS (Atkin, 1993; Monismith, Shute, St. Pierre, & Alles, 1984; Signorielli, 1993). Others have used posters and billboards to warn adolescents of the chances of

---

[63] In fact, however, health issues are quite rarely portrayed realistically. Since its primary function is to promote commercial products, television is only secondarily concerned with public health issues. Often TV programs portray health problems as individual concerns rather than social ones and they tend to avoid discussions which will deeply offend their viewers or their sponsors (Montgomery, 1990; Signoriella, 1993; Wallack, 1990).

contracting a sexually transmitted disease or becoming pregnant if they are sexually active (Strasburger, 1993).

The relative success of such health promotion campaigns, however, is not entirely clear. Researchers indicate that the surveyed adolescents were aware of having seen antismoking messages on television, remembered them, and reported worrying about the dangers of smoking (Monismith, Shute, St. Pierre, & Alles, 1984). More than half of the respondents who smoked stated that their exposure to these announcements made them want to stop smoking but data were not collected on their subsequent smoking behaviors (Monismith, Shute, St. Pierre, & Alles, 1984). Evaluations of other anti-smoking campaigns, however, indicate that the media were effective at preventing some adolescents from beginning to smoke and even stimulated the cessation of smoking in others (Flay, 1987; Worden, Flynn, Geller, Chen, Shelton, Secker-Walker, Solomon, Solomon, Couchey, & Constanza, 1984).

There is also evidence to suggest that the news media can be an effective vehicle for health-promotion (Donnerstein & Linz, 1995). Research concerning the disclosure to the media of AIDS and HIV infection by celebrities, for example, indicates that such information directly corresponded to marked increases in the number of individuals requesting HIV-antibody testing (Gellert, Weismuller, Higgins, & Maxwell, 1992). Figure 6.2 illustrates this pattern.

Researchers point out changing health-impacting behaviors and attitudes is more effective if the messages promoted are designed with their target audience in mind. Rather than emphasizing the goals of the sponsoring organization, effective campaign strategies are careful to take into account the perspective of the target audience in terms of their "attitudes, beliefs, motivations, health behavior, and needs" (Sullivan & Robinson, 1994: 84).

Successful health promotion campaigns involve exposing the audience to information surrounding the health threat, providing them with an understanding concerning the importance of the threat, their susceptibility to it, and an understanding concerning what role they can play in its prevention or treatment.[64] According to some researchers, mass media are most effective in the first part of this process--increasing the audience's awareness and knowledge of the health threat (Rogers & Storey, 1987; Sullivan & Robinson, 1994). Health promotion campaigns have also proven effective in stimulating interpersonal discussions which are generally more directly responsible for behavioral change (Sullivan & Robinson, 1994).

---

[64]   Campaigns which emphasize the efficacy of actions or treatments will be more effective than those which leave the viewer believing they have no control over the health problem (Sullivan & Robinson, 1994).

Increasing Use of Available Services

Often adolescents do not use the available health care services. The urgent need for outreach into the community to attract adolescents to health care facilities has been thoroughly discussed, while not much research has been done on *how* to encourage adolescents to visit health care facilities (Goon & Berger, 1989). In an attempt to acquaint adolescents and their parents with the health care facility in a nontraditional manner, some clinics provide opportunities such as a *Teens Health Nite Out* (Vernon & Seymore, 1987).

This bimonthly experience for teens and their parents combines social interaction with discussion of health issues. The researchers found that it increases familial communication in the home about health issues.

Various researchers have noted the positive effects of peer-directed discussion and support groups, the use of charismatic older students as teachers, the incorporation of media materials with similar-age peers, the use of peer counselors, and the inclusion of young people in the planning of health education efforts (Bonaguro, Rhonehouse, & Bonaguro, 1988; Brown & Fritz, 1988; DiClemente, 1989; Holund, 1990; Kisker, 1985; Millar, 1975; Rickert, Jay, & Gottlieb, 1991). Research indicates that social skills training and social pressures curricula work best with peer leaders, but other kinds of instruction may be effective with either adult or adolescent teachers (Perry, Telch, Killen, Burke, & Maccoby, 1983). This interaction may explain the one study cited by Bonaguro and his colleagues (1988), which concluded that a teacher-led session was more effective than a peer- or expert-led session. The effectiveness of the instructor will be determined, in part, by the topic and focus.

Relatively simple changes in the characteristics of health care services may make a big difference in their perceived acceptability and accessibility by teens. Office hours should be arranged to meet the needs of the adolescents and their families; the waiting rooms and facilities should include reading material of interest to adolescents as well as other patients. Because fewer adolescents than adults have ready access to a car, it is especially important that adolescent health care facilities be located close to their patients and to public transportation routes.

FIGURE 6.2:   Alternative-Test-Site (Anonymous) HIV-Antibody Testing in Orange County, California, from July 1985 through May 1992

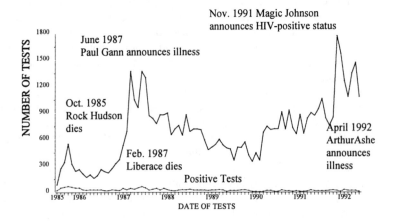

SOURCE: Gellert, Weismuller, Higgins, & Maxwell, 1994: Disclosure of AIDS in celebrities, Figure 4. *New England Journal of Medicine,* 327: 1389. Reprinted with permission.

Communication Between Health Care Providers, Patients, and Their Families

Once contact with an adolescent patient has been made, health careproviders must be careful to develop the most appropriate and effective patient/practitioner relationship. In light of the fact that this relationship is both important and potentially problematic, researchers have provided a number of useful suggestions to facilitate relationship development. First, most authors advocate a non-judgmental and nondirective communicative style (Arborelius & Bremberg, 1988; Friedman & Hedlund, 1991). The World Health Organization's training program for those who work with adolescents emphasizes such behaviors as attending skills, encouraging, reflecting, probing, and summarizing. Other suggestions include providing a minimal number of rules, consistency in enforcing the rules, focusing on responsibility to self, acknowledging the adolescent's frustrations, treating the teen with respect, and admitting mistakes (Rubin, 1986). Rules should be presented as facts of life--the care provider need not try to justify them--but artificial limit-setting should be avoided (Long, 1985).

A positive approach to working with the adolescent builds a "therapeutic alliance" in which the care provider allies with the adolescent's own efforts by identifying his or her strengths and goals (Long, 1985). Further communication is then related to these goals. Some researchers argue that the care provider should empathize with the teen without reinforcing delusions (Long, 1985; Vernon & Seymore, 1987). Practitioners should try to avoid criticizing the teen but provide direction which is clearly value-laden. A physician who seeks to promote sexual abstinence among young patients, for example, might develop the habit of asking each teen whether he has been able to "maintain his virginity" rather than if he "is sexually active."

Also, physicians and other practitioners should be aware that adolescents may have hidden agendas when they visit, and that it may even be useful to allow the adolescent to be vague about an original complaint (Vernon & Seymore, 1987). A secondary complaint may be used to gain access to a care provider, and the real issue may come out in discussion. As with any medical practice, continuity of care improves rapport, follow-up, and compliance. An effective practitioner will be able to gauge and adapt to the emotional state of the adolescent--an anxious teen needs support, while one who is more comfortable may be in a better position to confront realities (Long, 1985). Medical practitioners should be careful about accepting an adolescent's bravado as real.

Of particular help when communicating with adolescents may be metacommunication--discussion of the communication process. Research suggests that commenting on the interaction between the provider and the adolescent may open the relationship significantly (Long, 1985). Several other specific suggestions are available in the literature and can be incorporated into health communication efforts. Munger (1990) and Silber and Rosenthal (1986) report the effective use of a questionnaire regarding health concerns to be administered to adolescents upon their first visit to a health care facility. They find that such a questionnaire not only made care providers aware of concerns beyond the one that originally prompted the visit, but also provided the opening for discussion of the adolescents' concerns by helping to break the ice. The adolescents report feeling more comfortable initially responding to questions about health concerns on paper rather than orally.

Research also documents the utility of having fliers with information on health issues available, videotape presentations accompanying didactic lectures, and interactive software for adolescent acquisition of health information (Bosworth, Chewning, Day, Hawkins, & Gustafson, 1981; Kisker, 1985; Rickert, Gottlieb, & Jay, 1990). Even scare tactics or fear-appeals may have useful applications in regard to educating adolescents about health concerns, although sometimes they are counter productive (Brown & Fritz, 1988; Perry, Telch, Killen, Burke, & Maccoby, 1983). Explanations of health problems, health guidance, and treatment regimens will be more effective if they are in tune with an adolescent's developmental stage. Practitioners should consider a teenager's likely egocentricity as well as their feelings of invulnerability (Brown, & Fritz, 1988). To be consistent with the stages of adolescent development, messages targeted to younger adolescents should be concrete rather than abstract (Howard, 1985). An analysis of elements common to successful, rigorous programs indicated that the inclusion of information about immediate physiological effects, a discussion of resistance to peer, family, and media influences, and the use of multiple strategies should also be considered (Bonaguro, Rhonehouse, & Bonaguro, 1988). Overall, a health education program should provide a supportive environment that encourages participation and responsibility by the adolescent and his or her family (Bernard, 1986).

Research also indicates that, in terms of general health information, physicians place more emphasis on all topics than do teens, but physicians also underestimate the importance that adolescents place on almost all health topics. (Levenson, Pfefferbaum, & Morrow, 1987). This same inconsistency was noted when adolescent perceptions were compared with those of health teachers and school nurses (Levenson, Morrow, Morgan, & Pfefferbaum, 1986). While all groups rated sex, drugs, and the body as important topics, the adolescents also rated safety and fitness concerns highly. Focusing on pregnant teens, Levenson, Smith, and Morrow (1986) noted agreement between physicians and the teens on the importance of all health topics except birth control, which was rated much higher by physicians than it was by the already-pregnant teens. However, the physicians perceived that the teens did not think that any of the health topics were as important as the teens actually did. In particular, the adolescents desired more information about parenting, health dangers to the baby, and infant growth and development than the physicians perceived. No significant differences among physicians were noted (Levenson, Smith, & Morrow, 1986). This finding is an important one, because physicians may come across as condescending, overly solicitous, insensitive, or disrespectful if their perceptions of adolescent concerns are incorrect. Such perceptual differences may help, in part, to explain the finding that adolescents perceive health care providers as inattentive and unresponsive to their unique needs (Rogers & Elliott, 1989).

CHAPTER 7

GUIDELINES FOR MEETING THE CHALLENGE OF ADOLESCENT HEALTH IN A MORALLY CONSISTENT MANNER

Previous chapters have documented the health problems of adolescents, discussed the barriers and issues associated with providing health care to teens, and provided suggestions for improving health care delivery by overcoming barriers and addressing difficult social and moral issues. Earlier chapters also have discussed the social context in which adolescent health problems occur and articulated principles from Catholic moral and social teaching that form the basis for the development of guidelines relevant to adolescent health care.

This chapter provides general guidelines that can be used to develop, evaluate, and improve adolescent health care delivery. These guidelines integrate Catholic social and moral teaching with the principles underlying democratic communitarianism, including the sacredness of the individual, solidarity, complementary association, and participation (Bellah, 1994). They incorporate and generalize from the many specific suggestions for improving health care discussed in the previous chapter. Morally consistent adolescent health care should be value-based, family-centered, and integrated health care. It should emphasize prevention and early intervention, be culturally competent, and be responsive to age-specific needs and social pressures under which adolescents are developing.

VALUE-BASED HEALTH CARE

Adolescent health care should be anchored in the fundamental values of Catholic moral and social teaching which are universal precepts of many major religions.

1. Adolescent health care policies and programs must be based on the concept of human dignity.

2. Policies and programs must suggest the individual as a whole person including physical, psychological, social, and spiritual dimensions.

3. Policies and programs must respect individual rights and responsibilities but within familial and communal frameworks and in the context of the common good.

4. Policies and programs must address the interdependence between personal, familial, and societal responsibility for addressing adolescent health care needs.

5. Policies and programs must value life and discourage conditions that diminish human dignity. They must avoid any indication of support of culturally accepted behaviors and procedures which de-value human life and dignity including the use or distribution of contraception among unmarried teens, abortion, and the use of physical violence to settle disputes.

6. The health care system must adopt a preferential option for the poor which imposes a prophetic mandate to speak for those who have no one to speak for them: the poor. Appropriate policies to address the social and financial problems associated with the care of poor adolescents will enable these young people to help themselves.

CULTURALLY-COMPETENT HEALTH CARE

Providers of health care for adolescents should strive to value cultural diversity, recognize the inherent strengths of different cultural systems, and reduce the negative impact of their own biases as much as possible. Health care services should take into account the human dignity of all individuals and not discriminate on the basis of social and cultural characteristics.

1. Adolescent health care policies and programs, as well as individual care providers, must be sensitive to the values and beliefs of adolescents and families from diverse cultural backgrounds.

2. Policies and programs must strive to achieve ethnic, racial, gender, and cultural representation among providers proportional to the representation among users of the services and find the resources and ability to accommodate these differences in delivering health care.

3. Training and education of health care providers should include issues of cultural diversity: a development of respect for the culture of different groups; and an understanding of how these differences affect the culture of adolescents.

AGE-APPROPRIATE HEALTH CARE

Health care service providers should be attuned to age- and developmentally-specific needs of adolescents and to the social context within which teens make health-impacting decisions. They need to view each adolescent as a whole person developing in a broad social context that increases vulnerability to health-compromising behavior.

1. Adolescent health care policies and programs must take into account age- and developmentally-specific problems and needs, for example, privacy, communication, facility convenience, and youth-oriented staff.

2. Efforts should be made to reduce the promotion of health-compromising behaviors among young people in mass media. At the very least, the information concerning social morbidities and health-compromising behaviors which is propagated in mass media should be balanced with pro-social and health-improving information.

FAMILY-CENTERED HEALTH CARE

Adolescent health services should emphasize the importance of the family in the development and care of young people. Catholic teaching stresses the family as the foundation of the church, the society, and the community. This entails forging a partnership of society and families that seeks solutions to enable the health and well-being of adolescents.

1. Adolescent health care policies and programs must recognize, affirm, and support the integrity of the family unit.

2. Policies and programs must reinforce and enhance parents' primary and fundamental right and responsibility for their children's education, socialization, and health care. These policies and programs must also foster the developmentally appropriate transfer of these rights and responsibilities to the young adult.

3. Policies and programs must respond to the inability of some families to deal with their children's health problems adequately.

4. Policies and programs must address adolescent health care issues at the appropriate societal level. They should support the principle of subsidiarity and a family perspective by strengthening families, churches, neighborhoods, and other community organizations in the planning, development, and implementation of health care programs for adolescents.

PREVENTIVE HEALTH CARE

Adolescent health care should be oriented toward preventive and early intervention strategies. These strategies limit the severity and consequences of many health problems including biomedical and mental illnesses and social morbidities. Preventive care and early interventions also are associated with reduced costs.

1. Adolescent health care policies and programs must recognize the value of early and ongoing prevention that could avoid many of the difficulties that otherwise appear or become exacerbated during adolescence.

2. Policies and programs must focus on prevention efforts begun during childhood and early intervention begun in early adolescence when prevention is impossible or ineffective.

3. The church, service providers, health care organizations, families, and other individuals need to actively advocate for policy changes

promoting health in adolescents. Resources for preventative policies and programs need to be garnered through the efforts of such adults.

INTEGRATED COMMUNITY-BASED HEALTH CARE

Adolescent health care will be strengthened if the services, policies, and programs provided are integrated. Programs should be oriented to treating the whole person in the context of his/her family and community ties. The whole person includes physical, intellectual, emotional, social, and spiritual dimensions. Integrated health care also is designed to address the broad range of developmental and biopsychosocial needs of adolescents as well as the clustering of problems within individuals and families.

1. Adolescents and their families must have the knowledge and skills needed to participate in their own care and make responsible choices regarding health care, for example, how to prevent health problems and when and how to access the health-care system. When adolescents lack such skills, efforts should be made to promote educational programing addressing these needs.

2. Policies and programs must foster integrated, comprehensive, and intensive services that treat the whole person and take into account the social context of their varied environments, because so many adolescents experience multiple interrelated problems that can not be treated in isolation.

3. Policies and programs must provide opportunities for adolescents, families, schools, churches, neighborhood organizations and human services and health care providers to collaborate in the design, assessment, planning, and implementation of adolescent health care services.

4. Health care providers and practitioners, families, the church, and other organizations need to actively work for the removal of barriers to effective health care delivery to the adolescents in their communities and to locate and designate resources for their support.

5. Professionals engaged in health care delivery should receive training to encourage collaborative, multi-discipline, and integrated health care organizations.

BIBLIOGRAPHY

Aaron, H.J., Mann, T.E., & Taylor, T. (Eds.). 1994. *Values and public policy.* Washington, DC: The Brookings Institution.

A.C. Nielsen Company. 1993. *Nielsen report on television 1993.* Northbrook, IL: Nielsen Media Research.

Ackerman, G.L. 1993. A congressional view of youth suicide. *American psychologist -special issue on adolescence*, 48: 183-184.

Ad Hoc Committee on Marriage and Family Life, National Conference of Catholic Bishops. 1988. *A family perspective in church and society: a manual for all pastoral leaders.* Washington, DC: United States Catholic Conference.

Adamek, R.J., & Thoms, A.I. 1991. Responsible sexual values program: the first year. *Family Perspective*, 25: 67-81.

Adams, P.F., & Hardy, A.M. 1989. Current estimates from the national health interview survey, 1988. *Vital and Health Statistics, Series* 10, 173. Hyattsville, MD: National Center for Health Statistics.

Adelson, L. 1992. The gun and the sanctity of human life; or the bullet as pathogen. *Arch Surgery*, 127: 171-176.

Adger, H.J., McDonald, E.M., & Deangelis, C. 1990. Substance abuse education in pediatrics. *Pediatrics*, 86: 555-560.

Adler, N.E. 1992. Unwanted pregnancy and abortion: Definitional and research issues. *Journal of Social Issues*, 48: 19-35.

Adler, R.S., & Jellinek, M.S., 1990. After teen suicide: Issues for pediatricians who are asked to consult to schools. *Pediatrics*, 86: 982-987.

Adler-Stier, E. S., & Merdinger, J. M. 1990. Schools and systems: policies and programs for pregnant and parenting adolescents. In Arlene R. Stiffman and Ronald A. Feldman (Eds.). *Advances in adolescent mental health, Vol. 4*, pp. 173-188. London: Jessica Kingsley Publishers.

Adolescent Health Program, University of Minnesota. 1989. *Proceedings from the 1989 Adolescent Health Coordinators Conference in Denver, Colorado, August 8-10, 1989.* Washington, DC: National Center for Education in Maternal and Child Health.

Advance Data No. 99. 1984. *Health care of adolescents by office-based physicians: National ambulatory medical care survey,* 1980-1981. Washington, DC: National Center for Health Statistics.

Agranoff, R. 1981. City Manager's Human Service Committee, A city human services policy: The case of cincinnati. In Robert Agranoff (Ed.), *Human services on a limited budget*, pp. 81-90. Washington, DC: International City Management Association.

Agranoff, R. 1983. *Human services on a limited budget.* Washington, DC: International City Management Association.

Agranoff, R. 1991. Human services integration: Past and present challenges in public administration. *Public Administration Review*, 51: 533-542.

Ahn, N. 1994. Teenage childbearing and high school completion: Accounting for individual heterogeneity. *Family Planning Perspectives*, 26: 17-21.

Airhihenbuwa, C.O. 1989. *Health education for African Americans: A neglected task.* Health Education, 20: 9-14.

Alexander, E. 1990. School-based clinics: Questions to be answered in planning stages. *The High School Journal*, (Dec/Jan.): 133-138.

Allen, L., & Majidi-Ahi, S. 1990. Black American children. In Jewelle Taylor Gibbs, Larke Nahme Huang, and Associates (Eds.), *Children of color: Psychological interventions with minority youth*, pp. 148-178. San Francisco: Jossey-Bass Publishers.

Allen, M., Brown, P., & Finlay, B. 1992. *Helping children by strengthening families.* Washington, DC: Children's Defense Fund.

Allington, R.L., & Johnson, P. 1989. Coordination, collaboration, and consistency. In Robert E. Slavin, Nancy L. Karweit, and Nancy C. Madden (Eds.), *Effective programs for students at risk*, pp. 320-354. Boston, MA: Allyn and Bacon.

Alter, C., & Hage, J. 1993. *Organizations working together.* Newbury Park, CA: Sage Publications.

Althaus, F. 1994. Age at which young men initiate intercourse is tied to sex education and mother's presence in the home. *Family Planning Perspectives*, 26: 142-143.

Amaro, H., & Zuckerman, B. 1990. Patterns and prevalence of drug use among adolescent mothers. In Arlene R. Stiffman and Ronald A. Feldman (Eds.), *Adolescent mental health: a research-practice annual*, pp. 203-221. London: Jessica Kingsley Publisher

Ambuel, B.H. 1989. Developmental change in adolescents' psychological and legal competence to consent to abortion: An empirical study and quantitative model of social policy. *Dissertation Abstracts International,* pp. 3183-B.

Ambuel, B. H., & Rappaport, J. 1992. Developmental trends in adolescents' psychological and legal competence to consent to abortion. *Law and Human Behavior*, 16: 129-153.

American Academy of Pediatrics, Committee on Adolescence. 1990. *Sex education: A bibliography of educational materials for children, adolescents, and their families.* Elk Grove Village, IL: American Academy of Pediatrics, Division of Publications.

American Academy of Pediatrics. 1991a. American academy of pediatrics officials answer access proposal questions. *American Academy of Pediatrics News*, 7.

American Academy of Pediatrics. 1991b. *Children our future, American Academy of Pediatrics Conference for Media Proceedings.* Elk Grove Village, IL: American Academy of Pediatrics.

American Academy of Pediatrics. 1992a. Statement offers guidelines on school based clinics. *American Academy of Pediatrics News*, 8: 14-20.

American Academy of Pediatrics. 1992b. Study compares access proposals. *American Academy of Pediatrics*, 8: 4.

American College of Physicians. 1989. Health care needs of the adolescent. *Annals of Internal Medicine*, 110: 930-935.

American Family. 1993. Teenage pregnancy: Sex education v. Family planning. *American Family*, pp. 16.

American Medical Association. 1992. *Guidelines for adolescent preventive services*. Chicago, IL: American Medical Association.

American Medical Association Council on Scientific Affairs. 1989a. Health care needs of homeless and runaway youths. *Journal of the American Medical Association*, 262: 1358-1361.

American Medical Association Council on Scientific Affairs. 1989b. *Information report: Recognition of childhood sexual abuse as a factor in adolescent health issues*. Chicago, IL: American Medical Association.

American Medical Association Council on Scientific Affairs. 1989c. Providing medical services through school-based health programs. *Journal of the American Medical Association*, 261: 1939-1942.

American Medical Association Council on Scientific Affairs. 1993a. Adolescents as victims of family violence. *Journal of the American Medical Association*, 270: 1850-1856.

American Medical Association Council on Scientific Affairs. 1993b. Confidential health services for adolescents. *Journal of the American Medical Association*, 269: 1420-1424.

American Medical Association Council on Scientific Affairs. 1990. Health status of detained and incarcerated youths. *Journal of the American Medical Association*, 263: 987-991.

American Medical Association: Group on Science and Technology. 1994. Athletic preparticipation examinations for adolescents. *Archives of Pediatrics and Adolescent Medicine*, 148: 93-98.

American Public Welfare Association. 1986. *Investing in poor families and their children: A matter of commitment, Final Report Part I: One child in four*. Washington, DC: The American Public Welfare Association.

American Public Welfare Association. 1988. *Investing in poor families and their children: A matter of commitment: Access, Final Report Part II*. Washington, DC: The American Public Welfare Association.

American School Health Association, Association for Advancement of Health Education, & Society for Public Health Education Incorporated 1989. *The national adolescent student health survey: A report on the health of America's youth*. Oakland, CA: Third Party Publishing.

Amos, A. 1991. Young people, tobacco, and 1992. *Health Education Journal*, 50: 26-42.

Anderson, E. 1991. Neighborhood effects on teenage pregnancy. In Christopher Jencks and Paul E. Peterson (Eds.), *The urban underclass*, pp. 375-398. Washington, DC: Brookings.

Anderson, G.M. 1995. Gun control: New approaches. *America*, pp. 26-29.

Anderson, J.E., Freese, T.E., & Pennbridge, J.N. 1994. Sexual risk behavior and condom use among street youth in Hollywood. *Family Planning Perspectives*, 26: 22-25.

Anderson, R. M., Giachello, A. L., & Aday, L. A. 1986. Access of Hispanics to health care and cuts in services: A state-of-the-art overview. *Public Health Reports*, 101: 238-252.

Aral, S.O., Schaffer, J.E., Mosher, W.D., & Cates, W.J. 1988. Gonorrhea rates: What denominator is most appropriate? *American Journal of Public Health*, 78: 702-703.

Arboreilius, E., & Bremberg, S. 1988. It is your decision--Behavioral effects of a student-centered health education model at school for adolescents. *Journal of Adolescence*, 11: 287-297.

Arbuckle, G.A. 1986. Theology and anthropology: Time for dialogue. *Theological Studies*, 47: 428-447.

Archdiocese of Boston. 1986. *Report on school-based health clinics*. Boston, MA: Daughters of St. Paul.

Archdiocese of Cincinnati. 1986. Prelate seeks 'ironclad' assurance clinics won't peddle contraceptives. *Catholic Telegraph*, September 19, 1986.

Archdiocese of Denver. 1987. Parents urged to shun school clinics, pp. 1-3. Denver, CO: Pro-life Office, Office of Communications, Catholic Archdiocese of Denver.

Archdiocese of Los Angeles. 1986. Archbishop asks governor to halt abortion funding. Tidings.

Archdiocese of Miami. 1986. Birth control, schools don't mix: Statement of Florida Bishops on public school programs in human sexuality. *The Voice*, 2: 12-14.

Armacost, R.L. (Undated). *Evaluation and interpretation of pregnancy impact of six school-based clinics.* Unpublished paper, Marquette University.

Association of American Medical Colleges. 1993. Medical school admission requirements 1994-1995: United States and Canada. Washington, DC: Association of American Colleges.

Astone, N.M. 1993. Thinking about teenage childbearing. *Journal of the Institute for Philosophy and Public Policy.*

Atkin, C.K. 1993. Effects of media alcohol messages on adolescent audiences. In Victor C. Strasburger and George A. Comstock (Eds.). *Adolescent medicine: Adolescents and the media,* 4 (3): 527-542. Philadelphia: Hanley & Belfus, Inc.

Avison, W.R. & McAlpine, D.D. 1992. Gender differences in symptoms of depression among adolescents. *Journal of Health and Social Behavior*, 33: 77-96.

Bailey, L., Ginsburg, J., Wagner, P., Noyes, W., Christakis., G., & Dinning, J. 1982. Serum ferritin as a measure of iron stores in adolescents. *The Journal of Pediatrics*, 101: 774-775.

Balentine, M., Stitt, K.R., Bonner, J., & Clark, L.J. 1991. Self-reported eating disorders of African-American, low income adolescents: Behavior, body weight perceptions, & methods of dieting. *Journal of School Health*, 61: 392-396.

Bandini, L.G. 1992. Obesity in the adolescent. In Michael P. Nussbaum and Johanna T. Dwyer (Eds.), *Adolescent medicine: Adolescent nutrition and eating disorders*, 3 (3): 459-472. Philadelphia, PA: Hanley & Belfus, Inc.

Bandura, A. 1986. *The social foundations of thought and action.* Englewood Cliffs, NJ: Prentice-Hall.

Barbarin, O.A., & Tirado, M. 1985. Enmeshment, family processes, and successful treatment of obesity. *Family Relations*, 34: 115-121.

Barnard, C.A. 1990. *The long-term psychological effects of abortion.* Portsmouth, NH: Institute for Pregnancy Loss.

Barret, R.L., & Robinson, B.E. 1990. The role of adolescent fathers in parenting and childrearing. In Arlene R. Stiffman and Ronald A. Feldmen (Eds.), *Adolescent mental health: A research-practice annual*, pp. 189-200. London: Jessica Kingsley Publishers.

Bauman, K.E., Padgett, C.A., & Koch, G.G. 1989. A media-based campaign to encourage personal communication among adolescents about not smoking cigarettes: Participation, selection and consequences. Health Education Research, 4: 35-44.

Baumeister, A.A., Kupstas, F.D., & Klindworth, L.M. 1991. The new morbidity: A national plan of action. *American Behavioral Scientist*, 34(4): 468-500.

Baumrind, D. 1987. A developmental perspective on adolescent risk taking in contemporary America. In Charles E. Irwin, Jr. (Ed.), *Adolescent social behavior and health*, pp. 93-125. San Francisco, CA: Jossey-Bass.

Bayatpour, M., Wells, R. D., & Holford, S. 1992. Physical and sexual abuse as predictors of substance use and suicide among pregnant teenagers. *Journal of Adolescent Health*, 13: 128-132.

Bazron, B. 1989. *The minority severely emotionally disturbed child: considerations for special education and mental health services.* Washington, DC: CASSP Technical Assistance Center, Georgetown University Child Development Center.

Behrman, R., Vaughan, V.C., & Nelson, W.E. 1987. *Nelson's textbook of pediatrics*. Philadelphia: W.B. Saunders.

Bellah, R.N. 1996. "Families in the context of community" In P. Voydanoff (ed.), *Families and communities in partnership*, pp. . Lanham, MD: University Press of America.

Bellah, R.N., Madsen, R., Sullivan, W.M., Swidler, A., & Tipton, S.M. 1985. *Habits of the heart: Individualism and commitment in American life.* Berkeley, CA: University of California Press.

Benard, B. 1989. Working together: Principles of effective collaboration. *Prevention Forum*, 10: 4-9.

Benard, B. 1993. Fostering resiliency in kids. *Educational Leadership*, 51: 44-48.

Benda, B., & DiBlasio, T. 1991. Comparison of four theories of adolescent sexual exploration. *Deviant Behavior*, 12: 235-257.

Bensinger, J.S., & Nathenson, A.H. 1991. Difficulties in recognizing adolescent health issues. In William R. Hendee (Ed.), *The health of adolescents*, pp. 381-410. San Francisco, CA: Jossey-Bass.

Bernard, B. 1986. Characteristics of effective prevention programs. *Network*, 3: 6-8.

Bernardin, J. 1983. Call for a consistent life ethic. *Origins*, 13 (December 29): 491-494.

Bernardin, J. 1984. Enlarging the dialogue on a consistent ethic of life. *Origins*, 13 (April 5.

Bernardin, J. 1994. "The consistent ethic of life and health care reform." Address to the National Press Club, May 26, Washington, DC.

Berreth, D., & Scherer, M. 1993. *On transmitting values: A conversation with Amitai Etzioni*, 51: 12-15.

Besharov D. 1993a. It's time for common sense on using norplant. *The Philadelphia Inquirer*, Sunday May 23, 1993.

Besharov, D. 1993b. Norplant v. Abortion: A moral choice. *National Review*, August 9: 50-52.

Besharov, D. 1994. Risks and realism: Teen sex. In Jayne Garrison, Mark D. Smith, & Douglas J. Besharov (Eds.), *Sex education in the schools*, pp. 61-74. Menlo Park, CA: Henry J. Kaiser Family Foundation.

Besharov, D. J., & Gardiner, K. N. 1993. Truth and consequences teen sex: First of a two-part series. *The American Enterprise*, (Jan/Feb.): 52-59.

Bevilacqua, A. 1987. The question raised by school-based health clinics. *Origins*, 17: 187-190.

Bindman, A.B., Grumbach, K., Keane, D. Rauch, L., & Luce, J.M. 1991. Consequences of queuing for care at a public hospital emergency department. *Journal of the American Medical Association*, 266: 1091-1096.

Blau, G.M., & Gullotta, T.P. 1993. Promoting sexual responsibility in adolescence. In Thomas P. Gullotta, Gerald R. Adams, and Raymond Montemayor (Eds.), *Adolescent sexuality*, pp. 181-203. Newbury Park, CA: Sage Publications.

Blau, D.M., & Robins, P. K. 1991. Child care demand and labor supply of young mothers over time. *Demography*, 28: 333-351.

Blendon, R.J., & Edwards, J.N. 1991. Caring for the uninsured: Choices for reform. *Journal of the American Medical Association*, 265: 2563-2565.

Blum, B.B. 1990. *Five million children: A statistical profile of our poorest young citizens.* New York, NY: National Center for Children in Poverty.

Blum, R. 1987a. Contemporary threats to adolescent health in the United States. *Journal of the American Medical Association*, 257: 3390-3395.

Blum, R. 1987b. Physicians' assessment of deficiencies and desires for training in adolescent care. *Journal of Medical Education*, 62: 401-407.

Blum, R. 1988. Adolescent health. In Helen M. Wallace, George Ryan, and Allan C. Oglesby (Eds.), *Maternal and child health practices*, pp. 531-538. Oakland, CA: Third Party Publishing Company.

Blum, R. 1991. Global trends in adolescent health. *Journal of the American Medical Association*, 265: 2711-2719.

Blum, R., & Bearinger, L.H. 1990. Knowledge and attitudes of health professionals toward adolescent health care. *Journal of Adolescent Health Care*, 11: 289-294.

Blum, R.W., Resnick, M.D., & Stark, T. 1987. The impact of parental notification law on adolescent abortion decision-making. *American Journal of Public Health*, 77: 619-620.

Blumenkrantz, D.G. 1992. *Fulfilling the promise of children's services: Why primary prevention efforts fail and how they can succeed.* San Francisco, CA: Jossey-Bass Publishers.

Bolton, F.G. 1990. The risk of child maltreatment in adolescent parenting. In Arlene R. Stiffman and Ronald A. Feldman (Eds.), *Adolescent mental health: A research-practice annual Vol. 4*, pp. 223-237. London: Jessica Kingsley Publishers.

Bonaguro, J.A., Rhonehouse, M., & Bonaguro, E.W. 1988. Effectiveness of four school health education projects upon substance use, self-esteem, and adolescent stress. *Health Education Quarterly*, 15: 81-92.

Bosworth, K., Chewning, B., Day, T. Hawkins, R., & Gustafson, D. 1981. BARNEY: A computer based health information system for adolescents. *Journal of Early Adolescence*, 1: 315-321.

Boyer, C.B. 1990. Psychosocial, behavioral, and educational factors in preventing sexually transmitted diseases. In Manuel Schydlower and Mary-Ann Shafer (Eds.), *Adolescent Medicine: AIDS and other sexually transmitted diseases*, 1 (3): 597-613. Philadelphia, PA: Hanley & Belfus, Inc.

Boyer, D., & Fine, D. 1992. Sexual abuse as a factor in adolescent pregnancy and child maltreatment. *Family Planning Perspectives*, 24: 4-11.

Brady, S. 1993. Preventing hand gun violence: We must act now to save our kids. *NASSP Bulletin*, 4-8.

Brandt, R.S. 1986. On improving achievement of minority children: A conversation with James Comer. *Educational Leadership*, 43: 13-17.

Braverman, P. 1996. Herpes, syphilis, and other ulcerogenital conditions. In Paul G. Dyment (Ed.), *Adolescent medicine: Male reproductive health*, 7 (1): 93-118. Philadelphia, PA: Hanley & Belfus, Inc.

Brent, D., Perper, J., Allmam, C. Moritz, G., & Wartella, M. 1991. The presence and accessibility of firearms in the homes of adolescent suicide. *Journal of the American Medical Association*, 266: 2989-2995.

Brent, D.A., Perper, S.A., Goldstein, C.E., Kolko, D.J., Allan, M.J., Allman, C.J., & Zelenak, J.P. 1988. Risk factors for adolescent suicide. *Archives of General Psychiatry*, 45: 581-588.

Brick, P., & Roffman, D.M. 1993. "Abstinence, no buts" is simplistic. *Educational Leadership*, 51: 90-92.

Brindis, C. 1992. Adolescent pregnancy prevention for Hispanic youth: The role of schools, families, and communities. *Journal of School Health*, 62: 345-351.

Broihier, C.A. 1993. What about teen nutrition? *Current Health*, pp. 14-16.

Bronow, R., Beltran, R., Cohen, S. Elliot, P., Goldman, G., & Spotnitz, S. 1991. The physicians who care plan: Preserving quality and equitability in American medicine. *Journal of the American Medical Association*, 265: 2511.

Brookman, R. 1988a. Cocaine use: Medical consequences. *Adolescent Wellness Newsletter*, 1(Summer): 4-5.

Brookman, R. 1988b. Inhalants: A multifaceted problem. *Adolescent Wellness Newsletter*, 1(Fall): 4-5.

Brookman, R. 1989a. Menstrual and pelvic disorders. In Adele D. Hofmann and Donald E. Greydanas (Eds.), *Adolescent medicine*, pp. 371-382. Norwalk, CT: Appleton & Lange.

Brookman, R. 1989b. OTC and prescription drugs: Hidden dangers. *Adolescent Wellness Newsletter*, 1(Spring): 4-5.

Brooks, B.D., & Kann, M.E. 1993. What makes character education programs work? *Educational Leadership*, 51: 19-21.

Brooks, D., Smith, D., & Anderson, R. 1991. Medical apartheid: An American perspective. *Journal of the American Medical Association*, 266: 2746-2749.

Brooks-Gunn, J., Boyer, C., & Hein, K. 1988. Preventing HIV infection and AIDS in children and adolescents: Behavioral research and intervention strategies. *American Psychologist*, (Nov.): 958-964.

Brown, J.D., Greenberg, B.S., & Buerkel-Rothfuss, N.L. 1993. Mass media, sex, and sexuality. In Victor C. Strasburger and George A. Comstock, *Adolescent medicine: Adolescents and The media*, 4 (3): 511-526. Philadelphia: Hanley & Belfus, Inc.

Brown, L., & Fritz, G. 1988. AIDS education in the schools. *Clinical Pediatrics*, 27: 311-316.

Brown, R.T. 1993. Violence and adolescents. Unpublished lecture at Children's Medical Center, Dayton, OH: January 13, 1993.

Brown, R.T., & Coupey, S.M. 1993. Illicit drugs of abuse. In Manuel Schydlower and Peter Rogers (Eds.), *Adolescent medicine: Adolescent substance abuse and addictions*, 4: 321-340. Philadelphia, PA: Hanley & Belfus, Inc.

Brown, R.T., & Cromer, B.A. (Eds.). 1992. *Adolescent medicine: Psychosocial issues in adolescents*, 3 (1. Philadelphia: Hanley & Belfus, Inc.

Bruch, H.B. 1975. Emotional aspects of obesity in children. *Obesity: Pediatric Annals*, 91-99.

Bruner, C. 1991. *Thinking collaboratively: Ten questions & answers to help policy makers improve children's services.* Washington, DC: Education & Human Services Consortium, Institute for Educational Leadership.

Brunswick, A.F. 1988. Young black males and substance use. In Jewelle T. Gibbs, Ann F. Brunswick, Michael E. Connor, Richard Dembo, Tom E. Larson, Rodney J. Reed, and Barbara Solomon (Eds.), *Young, black, and male in America: An endangered species*, pp. 166-187. Dover, MA: Auburn House Publishing.

Bruvold, W.H. 1993. A meta-analysis of adolescent smoking prevention programs. *Journal of Public Health*, 83(June): 872-880.

Bryant, J., & Rockwell, S.C. 1994. Effects of massive exposure to sexually oriented prime-time television programming on adolescents' moral judgement. In Dolf Aillman, Jennings Bryant, and Althea C. Houston (Eds.). *Media, children and the family: Social scientific psychodynamic and clinical perspectives*, pp. 183-195. Hillsdale, NJ: Lawrence Erlbaum Associates.

Bulgar, R.J. 1993. Using academic health centers to help avoid health care's next crisis. *Journal of the American Medical Association*, 269: 2548-2549.

Bullock, W. 1992. Assessing burdens and benefits of medical care. *Origins*, 21: 553.

Bureau of Justice Statistics. 1992. *Criminal victimization in the United States 1990*. Washington, DC: Department of Justice, Office of Justice Programs, Bureau of Justice Statistics.

Burnhill, M.S. 1994. Adolescent pregnancy rates in the US. *Contemporary Pediatrics*. 11: 43-48.

Burt, M.R. 1990. Public costs and policy implications of teenage childbearing. In Arlene R. Stiffman and Ronald A. Feldman (Eds.), *Adolescent mental health: A research-practice annual*, pp. 265-280. London: Jessica Kingsley Publishers.

Bury, J.K. 1991. Teenage sexual behavior and the impact of AIDS. *Health Education Journal*, 50: 43-48.

Butler, S. 1991. A tax reform strategy to deal with the uninsured. *Journal of the American Medical Association*, 265: 2541-2544.

California Catholic Conference. 1987. *Parental primacy in the raising of children: Statement of the California Catholic Conference on school-based clinics*. California Catholic Conference.

Calista, D.J. 1986. Linking policy intention and policy implementation: The Role of the organization in the integration of human services. *Administration and Society*, 18: 263-286.

Callahan, C.M., & Rivara, F.P. 1992. Urban high school youth and handguns. *Journal of the American Medical Association*, 267: 38-42.

Callan, J.P. 1993. Underage drinking. *Journal of the American Medical Association*, 269: 1385.

Campbell, T.L. 1992. Family interventions in physical health. In Russell J. Sawa (Ed.), *Family health care*, pp. 213-226. Newbury Park, CA: Sage Publications.

Campbell, T.L., & Treat, D.J. 1990. The family's influence on health. In Robert E. Rakel (Ed.), *Textbook of Family practice*. Philadelphia: Saunders Press.

Carlson, B. E., Abagnale, S. & Flatow, E. 1993. Services for at-risk, pregnant, and parenting teenagers: A consortium approach. *Families in Society: The Journal of Contemporary Human Services*. (June): 375-380.

Carnegie Council on Adolescent Development. 1989. Turning points: Preparing American youth for the 21st Century. *Report of the Task Force on Education of Young Adolescents*. New York, NY: Carnegie Corporation.

Cartoff, V.G., & Klerman, L.V. 1986. Parental consent for abortion: Impact of the Massachusetts law. *American Journal of Public Health*, 76: 397-400.

Casey, R.J., & Berman, J.S. 1985. The outcome of psychotherapy with children. *Psychological Bulletin*, 98: 388-397.

Casper, L. 1990. Does family interaction prevent adolescent pregnancy? *Family Planning Perspectives*, 22: 109-114.

Cassata, M., Skill, T., & Boadu, S.O. 1983. Life and death in the daytime television serial: A content analysis. In Mary Cassata and Thomas Skill (Eds.), *Life on daytime television: Tuning-in American serial drama*. Norwood, NJ: Ablex Publishing Corp.

Cates, W. 1990. The epidemiology and control of sexually transmitted diseases. In Manuel Schydlower and Mary-Ann Shafer (Eds.), *Adolescent medicine: AIDS and other sexually transmitted diseases*, 1 (3): 409-427. Philadelphia, PA: Hanley & Belfus, Inc.

Catholic Church. 1976. *Rites of the catholic church*. New York, NY: Pueblo Publishing Company.

Catholic Health Association. 1986. *No room in the marketplace: The health care of the poor*. St. Louis, MO: Catholic Health Association.

Catholic Health Association. 1991. *With justice for all?* St. Louis, MO: Catholic Health Association.

Catholic Health Association. 1992. *Setting relationships right: A working proposal for systemic healthcare reform.* St. Louis, MO: Catholic Health Association of the United States.

Catholic Health Association. 1993. *Setting relationships right: A proposal for systemic healthcare reform.* St. Louis, MO: Catholic Health Association of the United States.

Cella, D.F., Tulsky, D.S., Sarafin, B., & Thomas, C.R. 1992. Culturally relevant smoking prevention for minority youth. *Journal of School Health,* 62: 377-380.

Center for the Future of Children. 1992a. *Future of children: School-linked services.* Los Altos, CA: David and Lucile Packard Foundation.

Center for the Future of Children. 1992b. *The future of children: U.S. health care for children.* Los Altos, CA: David and Lucille Packard Foundation.

Center for the Study of Family Development. 1990. *A working draft for the teen health task group of the new futures board.* Dayton, OH: University of Dayton.

Center for the Study of Family Development. 1991. *Summary of Catholic literature on school-based health clinics.* Dayton, OH: University of Dayton.

Center for the Study of Social Policy. 1993. *Kids count data book: State profiles of child well-being.* Washington, DC: Center for the Study of Social Policy.

Centers for Disease Control. 1992. Physical fighting among high school students--United States, 1990. *Journal of the American Medical Association,* 267: 19-20.

Centers for Disease Control. 1993. Minors' access to tobacco--Missouri and Texas. *Journal of the American Medical Association,* 269: 1362-1364.

Cervera, N.J. 1993. Decision making for pregnant adolescents: Applying reasoned action theory to research and treatment. *Families in Society: The Journal of Contemporary Human Services,* June: 355-365.

Chafee, J.H. 1992. It's Time to Control Handguns. *Public Welfare,* Fall: 18-22.

Chamberlin, R.W. 1993. The "new morbidity": Behavioral problems of preschoolers. In Robert J. Haggerty, Klaus J. Roghmann, and Ivan B. Pless (Eds.), *Child health and the community*, pp. 95-117. New Brunswick, NJ: Transaction Publishers.

Chamie, M., Eisman, S., Forrest, J.D., Orr, M.T., & Torres, A. 1982. Factors affecting adolescents' use of family planning clinics. *Family Planning Perspectives*, 14: 126-139.

Chang, G., & Astrachan, B. 1988. The emergency department surveillance of alcohol intoxication after motor vehicle accidents. *Journal of the American Medical Association*, 260: 2533-2536.

Chang, G., Warner, V., & Weissman, M.M. 1988. Physicians' recognition of psychiatric disorders in children and adolescents. *American Journal of Diseases of Children*, 142: 736-739.

Chassin, L., Presson, C.C., Sherman, S.S., & Edwards, D.A. 1990. The natural history of cigarette smoking predicting young-adult smoking outcomes from adolescent smoking patterns. *Health Psychology*, 9: 701-716.

Cheng, T.L., Savageau, J.A., Sattler, A.L., & DeWitt, T.G. 1993. Confidentiality in health care: A survey of knowledge, perceptions, and attitudes among high school students. *Journal of the American Medical Association*, 269: 1404-1407.

Chi, K.S. 1987. What has happened to the comprehensive human services agency? *New England Journal of Human Services*, 7: 24-30.

Children's Defense Fund. 1989. *Lack of health insurance makes a difference.* Washington, DC: Children's Defense Fund.

Children's Defense Fund. 1990. *Latino youths at a crossroads.* Washington, DC: Children's Defense Fund.

Children's Defense Fund. 1991. *The state of America's children 1991.* Washington, D.C.: Children's Defense Fund.

Children's Defense Fund. 1992. *Helping children by strengthening families.* Washington, DC: Children's Defense Fund.

Children's Defense Fund. 1994. *The state of America's children yearbook 1994.* Washington, DC: Children's Defense Fund.

Children, Family, Drugs, and Alcoholism Subcommittee, Committee on Labor and Human Resources, & U.S. Senate 1991. *Behind closed doors: Family violence in the home. A hearing before the Subcommittee on Children, Family, Drugs, and Alcoholism, of the Committee on Labor and Human Resources.* Washington, DC: U.S. Government Printing Office.

Christian, W.P., & Larsson, E.V. 1992. Chapter 94: Legal issues. In Levine, Carey and Crocker (Eds.) *Developmental Behavioral Pediatrics*, pp. 771-781.

Christoffel, K.K. 1995. Foreword. In Katherine Kaufer Christoffel & Carol W. Runyan (Eds.), *Adolescent medicine: Adolescent injuries: Epidemiology and prevention*, 6 (2): *ix-x*. Philadelphia, PA: Hanley & Belfus, Inc.

Christopher, F.S., & Roosa, M.W. 1990. An evaluation of an adolescent pregnancy prevention program: Is "just say no" enough? *Family Relations*, 39: 68-72.

Claista, D.J. 1986. Linking policy intention and policy implementation: The role of the organization in the integration of human services. *Administration and Society*, 18: 263-286.

Clark, A.M., Thomson, H.D., Mantell, C.D., & Hutton, J.D. 1986. Comprehensive antenatal care and education of young adolescents: Beneficial effects on pregnancy and outcome. *New England Medical Journal*, 99: 59-62.

Clarke, T. 1980. *Above every name: The lordship of Christ and social systems.* New York, NY: The Paulist Press.

Clarke-Stewart, A., & Koch, J.B. 1983. *Children: Development through adolescence.* New York, NY: John Wiley & Sons.

Clayton, S. 1991. Gender differences in psychological determinants of adolescent smoking. *Journal of School Health*, 61: 115-120.

Cohall, A.T. & Cohall, R.M. 1995. "Number one with a bullet" Epidemiology and prevention of homicide among adolescents and young adults. In Katherine Kaufer Christoffel & Carol W. Runyan (Eds.), *Adolescent medicine: Adolescent injuries: Epidemiology and prevention*, 6 (2): 183-198. Philadelphia, PA: Hanley & Belfus, Inc.

Cohall, A.T., Cullins, V.E., Darney, P.D., & Nelson, A.L. 1993. Contraception in the 1990s: New methods and approaches. *Patient Care*. Moderator Andrea M. Kielich.

Coleman, E. 1982. Family intimacy and chemical abuse: The connection. *Journal of Psychoactive Drugs*, 14: 153-158.

Combs-Orme, T. 1993. Health effects of adolescent pregnancy: Implications for social workers. *Families in Society: The Journal of Contemporary Human Services*, (June): 344-354.

Comer, J.P. 1993. Inner-city education: A theoretical and intervention model. In W. J. Wilson (Ed.), *Sociology and the public agenda*. Newbury Park, CA: Sage Publications.

Comerci, G.D. 1988. Working with parents and adolescents: Negotiating a contract. *Adolescent Wellness Newsletter*, 1 (3): 2.

Comerci, G.D. 1989. Working with parents and adolescents: Developing effective support programs. *Adolescent Wellness*, (Spring): 2-3.

Comerci, G.D. 1991. Parents and society: How much the problem; How much the solution? In George D. Comerci and William A. Daniel (Eds.), *Adolescent medicine: Parenting the adolescent: Practitioner concerns*, 2 (2): 251-264. Philadelphia, PA: Hanley & Belfus, Inc.

Comerci, G.D. 1992. Eating disorders: Anorexia and bulimia. In Melvin D. Levine, William B. Carey, and Allen C. Crocker (Eds.), *Developmental-behavioral pediatrics*, pp. 364-369. Philadelphia, PA: W.B.Saunders Company.

Comerci, G.D., Brookman, R., Coupey, S., Ehrhardt, A., Sanders, J., & Whitaker, A. 1989. *Adolescent sexuality monograph: Adolescent wellness*. Lyndhurst, NJ: American Academy of Pediatrics.

Comerci, G.D., Brookman, R., Coupey, S., Sanders, J., & Shaffer, D. 1988a. *Alcohol/substance abuse monograph: Adolescent wellness*. Lyndhurst, NJ: American Academy of Pediatrics.

Comerci, G.D., Brookman, R., Coupey, S. Sanders, J., & Shaffer, D. 1988b. *Depression/suicide monograph: Adolescent wellness*. Lyndhurst, NJ: American Academy of Pediatrics.

Committee for Economic Development. 1987. *Children in need: Investment strategies for the educationally disadvantaged*. New York: Committee for Economic Development.

Committee for Economic Development. 1991. *The unfinished agenda: A new vision for child development and education*. New York: Committee for Economic Development.

Committee on School Health of the American Academy of Pediatrics. 1993. *School health: Policy and practice.* Elk Grove Village, IL: American Academy of Pediatrics.

Committee on School Health of the American Academy of Pediatrics & Newton, J. (Ed.), 1987. *School health: A Guide for health professionals.* Elk Grove Village, IL: American Academy of Pediatrics.

Comstock, G.A., & Strasburger, V.C. 1993. Media violence: Q & A. In Victor C. Strasburger and George A. Comstock (Eds.a. *Adolescent medicine: Adolescents and the media,* 4 (3): 495-510. Philadelphia: Hanley & Belfus, Inc.

Congressional Budget Office. 1993. *Managed competition and its potential to reduce health spending.* Washington, DC: U.S. Government Printing Office.

Congressional Budget Office. 1994. *An analysis of the administration's health proposal.* Washington, DC: U.S. Government Printing Office.

Connecticut Catholic Conference. 1987. *Concerning public school health clinics: A Statement by the catholic bishops of connecticut.* Conference Call, (Winter): 3-5.

Conrad, P., & Schneider, J. 1980. *Deviance and medicalization from badness to sickness.* St. Louis, MO: The C.V. Mosky Company.

Consortium of Family Organizations. 1992a. *Principles of family-centered health care.* Washington, DC: Consortium of Family Organizations.

Consortium of Family Organizations. 1992b. Principles of family-centered health care: A health care reform white paper. *Family Policy Report,* 2.

Consumer Reports. 1989. Can you rely on condoms? Consumer Reports, pp. 135-141

Cooke, G.J. 1993. Introduction: Focus on adolescent health: A call for action. *NAASP Bulletin,* 77: 1-3.

Cooperative Extension, University of Massachusetts, United States Department of Agriculture and Massachusetts Counties Cooperating. 1990. *Building communities of support for families in poverty.*

Corbett, T. 1991. *Coordination: A view from the streets.* Background Paper Prepared for the National Commission for Employment Policy Project on Coordination of Public Assistance Programs.

Costello, E.J., Edelbrock, C., Costello, A.J., Dulcan, M.K., Burns, B.J., & Brent, D. 1988. Psychopathology in pediatric primary care: The new hidden morbidity. *Pediatrics*, 82: 415-424.

Council on Scientific Affairs, American Medical Association. 1993. Adolescents as victims of family violence. *Journal of American Medical Association*, 270: 1850-1856.

Coupey, S.M. 1988. Infection in adolescents: Chlamydia. *Adolescent Wellness Newsletter Volume I* (Fall): 6-7. Lyndhurst, N.J.: Health Learning Systems Inc.

Coupey, S.M. 1989. Suicide risk among special groups of adolescents. *Adolescent Wellness Newsletter Volume I*, (Spring). Lyndhurst, NJ: Health Learning Systems Inc.

Coupey, S.M. 1992. Anorexia nervosa. In Stanford B. Friedman, Martin Fisher, and S. Kenneth Schonberg (Eds.), *Comprehensive adolescent health care*, pp. 217-231. St. Louis, MO: Quality Medical Publishing, Inc.

Coupey, S.M., & Klerman, L. (Eds.). 1992. Preface. *Adolescent medicine: Adolescent sexuality: Preventing unhealthy consequences*, 3 (2): 9-12. Philadelphia, PA: Hanley & Belfus, Inc.

Crisp, A.H. 1985. Gastrointestinal disturbance in anorexia nervosa. *Postgraduate Medical Journal*, 61: 3-5.

Cromer, B.A. 1992. Access to psychosocial care for adolescents. In Robert T. Brown and Barbara A. Cromer (Eds.). *Adolescent medicine: Psychosocial issues in adolescents*, 3 (1): 29-50. Philadelphia: Hanley & Belfus, Inc.

Cross, T., Bazran, B., Dennis, D., & Isaacs. 1989. *Towards a culturally competent system of care: A monograph on effective services for minority children who are severely emotionally disturbed.* Washington, DC: CASSP Technical Assistance Center.

Crum, G., & McCormack, T. 1992. *Abortion: Pro-choice or pro-life?* Washington, DC: The American University Press.

Crutcher, D. 1991. Family support in the home: Home visiting and public law 99-457: A Parent's Perspective. *American Psychologist*, 46: 138-140.

Cuellar, R.E., & Van Thiel, D.H. 1986. Gastrointestinal consequences of the eating disorders: Anorexia nervosa and bulimia. *The American Journal of Gastroenterology*, 81: 1113-1124.

Culhane, C. 1993. Report shows continued poor health habits in youth. *American Medical News*, 36(40): 11.

Cypress, B.K. 1984. Health care of adolescents by office-based physicians: National ambulatory medical care survey, 1980-81. *Advance Data from Vital and Health Statistics* No. 99. Hyattsville, M.D.: Public Health Service, DHHS.

Davies, J. 1991. Adolescent subculture. In Donald Ratcliff and James A. Davies (Eds.), Handbook of youth ministry, pp. 7-41. Birmingham, AL: R.E.P. Books.

Davis, K. 1991. Expanding medicare and employer plans to achieve universal health insurance. *Journal of the American Medical Association*, 265: 2525-2528.

Dawson, D. 1991. Family structure and children's health and well-being: Data from the 1988 National Health Interview Survey on Child Health. *Journal of Marriage and the Family*, 53: 573-584.

Dayton Daily News. 1993. Disease center undertakes study of teen violence, Wednesday, July 14, 1993.

DeJong, W., & Winsten, J.A. 1990. The use of mass media in substance abuse prevention. *Media and Substance Abuse*, pp. 30-46.

Demetriou, E., & Kaplan, D. 1989. Adolescent contraception use and parental notification. *American Journal of the Diseases of Children*, 143: 1166-1172.

De Pietro, R., & Clark, N. 1984. A sense-making approach to understanding adolescents' selection of health information sources. *Health Education Quarterly*, 11: 419-430.

De Veber, L.L., Ajzenstat, J., & Chisholm, D. 1991. Postabortion grief: Psychological sequelae of induced abortion. *Humane Medicine*, 7: 203-209.

Deschamps, I., Giron, B.J., & Lestradet, H. 1977. Blood glucose, insulin, and free fatty acid levels during oral glucose tolerance tests in 158 obese children. *Diabetes*, 26: 89-93.

Devine, C.M., Olson, C.M., & Frongillo, E.A. Jr. 1992. Impact of the nutrition for life program on junior high students in New York State. *Journal of School Health*, 62: 381-385.

DiClemente, R. 1989. Prevention of human immunodeficiency virus infection among adolescents: The interplay of health education and public policy in the development and implementation of school-based AIDS Education programs. *AIDS Education and Prevention*, 1: 70-78.

DiClemente, R., Boyer, C., & Mills, S. 1987. Prevention of AIDS among adolescents: Strategies for the development of comprehensive risk-reduction health education programs. *Health Education Research*, 2: 287-291.

Dietz, W.H. 1993. Television, obesity, and eating disorders. In Victor C. Strasburger and George A. Comstock (Eds.). *Adolescent medicine: Adolescents and the media*, 4 (3): 543-550. Philadelphia: Hanley & Belfus, Inc.

Dietz, W.H., & Gortmaker, S.L. 1993. TV or not TV: Fat is the question. *Pediatrics*, 91: 499-500.

Dietz, W.H., Gross, W.L., & Kirkpatrick, J.A. 1982. Blount disease (tibia vara): Another skeletal disorder associated with childhood obesity. *Clinical and Laboratory Observations*, 101: 735-737.

Dietz, W.H., & Strasburger, V.C. 1991. Children, adolescents, and television. *Current Problems in Pediatrics*, pp. 8-31.

Dodge, K., Bates, J., & Pettit, G. 1990. Mechanisms in the cycle of violence. *Science*, 250: 1678-1683.

Doherty, W.J. 1985. Family interventions in health care. *Family Relations*, 34: 129-137.

Doherty, W.J. 1992. Linkages between family theories and primary health care. In Russell J. Sawa (Ed.). *Family health care*, pp. 30-39. Newbury Park, CA: Sage Publications.

Doherty, W.J., & Campbell, T.J. 1988. *Families and health*. Beverly Hills, CA: Sage Publications Inc.

Doherty, W.J., & McCubbin, H.I. 1985. Families and health care: An emerging arena of theory, research, and clinical intervention. *Family Relations*, 34: 5-11.

Doll, W. 1984. Cooperation in Cleveland: Active partnerships between churches and foundations form an exemplary combination for serving the city's needs. *Foundation News*, (September/October): 66-71.

Donnelly, B.W., 1992. Chance to Grow: project evaluation. Unpublished report submitted to the Office of Adolescent Pregnancy Programs, Department of Health and Human Services.

Donnelly, B.W., & Davis-Berman, J., 1994. A review of the Chance to Grow Project: A care project for pregnant and parenting adolescents. *Child and Adolescent Social Work Journal*, 11: 493-506.

Donnerstein, E. & Linz, D. 1995. The mass media: A role in injury causation and prevention. In Katherine Kaufer Christoffel & Carol W. Runyan (Eds.), *Adolescent medicine: Adolescent injuries: Epidemiology and prevention*, 6 (2): 271-284. Philadelphia, PA: Hanley & Belfus, Inc.

Donovan, J.E., & Jessor, R. 1985. Structure of problem behavior in adolescence and young adulthood. *Journal of Consulting and Clinical Psychology*, 53: 890-904.

Dorr, D. 1983. *Option for the poor: A hundred years of vatican social teaching.* New York: Maryknoll.

Dougherty, D.M. 1993. Adolescent health: Reflections on a report to the US Congress. *American Psychologist - Special Issue on Adolescence*, 48: 193-201.

Doyle, D.M. 1988. What does god have to do with it? The meaning of AIDS. *Commonweal*, (June): 343-346.

Drogin, B. 1985. 'Got no choice' true victims of poverty: The children. *Los Angeles Times*, July 30, Part 1 page 1.

Dryfoos, J.G. 1988. School based clinics. In Helen M. Wallace, George Ryan, and Allan C. Oglesby (Eds.), *Maternal and child health practices*, pp. 563-571. Oakland CA: Third Party Publishing Company.

Dryfoos, J.G. 1990a. A review of interventions to prevent pregnancy. In Arlene R. Stiffman and Ronald A. Feldmen (Eds.), *Adolescent mental health: research-practice annual*, pp. 121-135. London: Jessica Kingsley Publishers.

Dryfoos, J.G. 1990b. *Adolescents at risk: Prevalence and prevention.* New York: Oxford University Press.

Dryfoos, J.G., & Klerman, L.V. 1988. School-based clinics: Their role in helping students meet the 1990 objectives. *Health Education Quarterly*, 15: 71-80.

Duncan, G.J., & Hoffman, S.D. 1991. Teenage underclass behavior and subsequent poverty: Have the rules changed? In Christopher Jencks and Paul E. Peterson (Eds.), *The urban underclass*, pp. 155-174. Washington DC: The Brookings Institution.

DuRant, R.H. 1991. Overcoming barriers to adolescents' access to health care. In William R. Hendee (Ed), *The health of adolescents*, pp. 431-452. San Francisco, CA: Jossey-Bass.

DuRant, R.H., Sanders, J.M., Jay, S. & Levinson, R. 1990. Adolescent contraceptive risk-taking behavior. In Arlene R. Stiffman and Ronald A. Feldmen (Eds.), *Adolescent mental health: Research-practice annual*, pp. 87-106. London: Jessica Kingsley Publishers.

Dwyer, J.T. 1992. Great expectations: Overview of adolescent nutrition for the year 2000 and beyond. In Michael P. Nussbaum and Johanna T. Dwyer (Eds.), *Adolescent medicine: Adolescent nutrition and eating disorder* 3 (3): 377-390. Philadelphia, PA: Hanley & Belfus, Inc.

Earls, F., Robins, L.N., Stiffman, A.R., & Powell, J. 1989. Comprehensive health care for high-risk adolescents: An evaluation study. *American Journal of Pediatric Health*, 79: 999-1005.

Eccles, J.S., Midgley, C., Wigfield, A., Miller-Buchanan, C.M., Reuman, D., Flanagan, C., & MacIver, Douglas 1993. Development during adolescence: The impact of stage-environment fit on young adolescent's experiences in schools and in families. *American Psychologist - Special Issue on Adolescence*, 48: 90-101.

Edelman, M.W. 1987. Preventing adolescent pregnancy. *Families in peril: An agenda for social change*. Cambridge, MA: Harvard University Press.

Edelman, P.B., & Radin, B.A. 1991. Serving children and families effectively: How the past can help chart the future. *The Education and Human Services Consortium*, 2-22.

Edwards, S. 1992. Sexually active adolescents have less knowledge and less fear of HIV than their abstinent peers. *Family Planning Perspectives*, 24: 142-143.

Edwards, S. 1994. As adolescent males age, risky behavior rises but condom use decreases. *Family Planning Perspectives*, 26: 45-46.

Eisen, M., Zellman, G.L., & McAlister, A. 1990. Evaluating the impact of a theory-based sexuality and contraceptive education program. *Family Planning Perspectives*, 22: 261-271.

Ekstrom, R.R. 1986. Youth culture and teen spirituality: signs of the times. In John Roberto (Ed.), *Readings in youth ministry: Foundations*, pp. 43-75. Washington, DC: National Federation for Cahtolic Youth Ministry.

Elder, J.P., & Stern, R.A. 1986. The ABCs of adolescent smoking prevention: An environment and skills model. *Health Education Quarterly*, 13: 181-191.

Elder, J.P., Wildey, M., de Moor, C., Sallis, J.F., Eckhardt, L., Edwards, C., Erickson, A., Golbeck, A., Hovell, M., Johnston, D., Levitz, M.D., Molgaard, C., Young, R., Vito, D., & Woodruff, S. 1993. The long-term prevention of tobacco use among junior high school students: Classroom & telephone interventions. *American Journal of Public Health*, 83(September): 1239-1244.

Elders, M.J., & Hui, J., 1992. Comprehensive school health services: Does It matter and is it worth the fight? *Ensuring student success through collaboration: summer institute papers and recommendations of the Council of Chief State School Officers.* Washington, DC: Council of Chief State School Officers.

Elders, M.J., & Hui, J. 1993. Making a difference in adolescent health. *Journal of the American Medical Association*, 269: 1425-1426.

Elkind, D. 1992. Cognitive development. In Stanford B. Friedman, Martin Fisher, and S. Kenneth Schonberg (Eds.), *Comprehensive adolescent health care*, pp. 24-26. St. Louis, MO: Quality Medical Publishing, Inc.

Ellers, B. 1993. Involving and supporting family and friends. In Margaret Gerteis, Susan Edgman-Levitan, Jennifer Daley, and Thomas L. Delbanco (Eds.), *Through the patient's eyes* pp. 178-203. San Francisco, CA: Jossey-Bass Publishers.

Ellickson, P.L., & Bell, R.M. 1990. Drug prevention in junior high: A multi-site longitudinal test. *Science*, (March) 247: 1299-1305.

Elster, A.B. 1990. Intervention models for promoting the parental behavior of adolescent mothers. In Arlene R. Stiffman and Ronald A. Feldman (Eds.), *Adolescent mental health: A research-practice annual*, 4: 161-171. London: Jessica Kingsley Publishers.

Elster, A.B., & Kuzsets, N.J. 1993. *Guidelines for adolescent preventive services* (GAPS). Baltimore, MD: Williams & Wilkins.

Elster, A.B., & Kuznets, N.J., 1994. *AMA guidelines for adolescent preventive services (GAPS): Recommendations and rationale.* Baltimore, MD: Williams & Wilkins.

Emery, K.J. 1994. Teen pregnancy prevention: What we know tells us what we should do. *Ohio Children*, pp. 4-5.

Enthoven, A.C. 1991. Market forces and health care costs. *Journal of the American Medical Association*, 266: 2751-2752.

Enthoven, A., & Kronick, R. 1991. Universal health insurance through incentives reform. *Journal of the American Medical Association*, 265: 2532-2536.

Escobedo, L.G., Marcus, S.E., Holtzman, D., & Giovino, G.A. 1993. Sports participation, age at smoking initiation, and the risk of smoking among U.S. high school students. *Journal of the American Medical Association*, 269: 1391-1395.

Evaluating Comprehensive Family Service Programs. 1992. Evaluating comprehensive family service programs. *Focus*, 14: 10-34.

Fabrega, H., 1981. Culture, biology and the study of disease. In Henry Rothschild (Ed.), *Biocultural aspects of disease,* pp. 54-94. New York, NY: Academic Press.

Fein, R. 1991. The Health security partnership: A federal-state universal insurance and cost-containment program. *Journal of American Medical Association*, 265: 2555-2558.

Feinstein, J.S. 1993. The relationship between socio-economic status and health: A review of the literature. *The Milbank Quarterly*, 71: 279-323.

Feldman, J. 1991. Commission issues access recommendations. *AAP News*, (August) 7: 1.

Feldman, S., & Elliott, R. 1990. *At the threshold: The developing adolescent.* Cambridge, MA: Harvard University Press.

Felice, M.E. 1992. Adolescence. In Melvin D. Levine, William B. Carey, and Allen C. Crocker (Eds.), *Developmental-behavioral pediatrics*, pp. 65-73. Philadelphia, PA: W.B.Saunders Company.

Fibkins, W.L. 1993. A program that worked: Combating student tobacco addiction in secondary schools. *NASSP Bulletin*, 77: 51-59.

Fiese, B.H. 1993. Family rituals in alcoholic and nonalcoholic households: Relations to adolescent health symptomology and problem drinking. *Family Relations*, 42: 187-192.

Fine, G.A., & Christoforides, L. 1991. Dirty birds, filthy immigrants, and the english sparrow war: Metaphorical linkage in constructing social problems. *Symbolic Interaction*, 14: 375-393.

Fingerhut, L.A., Ingram, D.D., & Feldman, J.J. 1992a. Firearm homicide among black teenage males in metropolitan counties: Comparison of Death rates in two periods, 1983 through 1985 and 1987 through 1989. *Journal of the American Medical Association*, 267: 54-58.

Fingerhut, L.A., Ingram, D.D., & Feldman, J.J. 1992b. Firearm and nonfirearm homicide among persons 15 through 19 years of age. *Journal of the American Medical Association*, 267: 48-53.

Fingerhut, L.A., & Kleinman, J.C. 1989. Trends in current status in childhood mortality United States, 1900-85. *Vital & Health Statistics Series 3*. Hyattsville, MD: National Center for Health Statistics.

Fingerhut, L.A., & Kleinman, J.C. 1990. International and interstate comparisons of homicide among young males. *Journal of the American Medical Association*, 263: 3292-3295.

Finkelhor, D. 1987. The sexual abuse of children: Current research review. *Psychiatric Annals*, 4: 233-241.

Finkelhor, D., Sedlak, A., & Hotaling, G. 1990. *Missing, abducted, runaway, and thrownaway children in America: First report, numbers and characteristics of national incidence studies: Executive summary.* Washington, DC: U.S. Department of Justice.

Fisher, M. 1992. Medical complications of anorexia and bulimia nervosa. In Michael P. Nussbaum and Johanna T. Dwyer (Eds.), *Adolescent medicine: adolescent nutrition and eating disorder* 3 (3): 487-502. Philadelphia, PA: Hanley & Belfus, Inc.

Fisher, M., Juszczak, L., Schneider, M., & Chapar, G. 1992. School-based adolescent health care. *American Journal of the Diseases of Children*, 146: 615-621.

Fishman, K.D. 1991. Therapy for Children. *The Atlantic Monthly*, (June): 47-81.

Fitzpatrick, S.B., Chacko, M.R., & Heald, F.P. 1984. Iron deficiency in black females during late adolescence. *Journal of Adolescent Health Care*, 5: 71-74.

Fitzpatrick, S.B., Fujii, C., Shragg, G.P., Rice, L., Morgan, M., & Felice, M. 1990. Do health care needs of indigent Mexican-American, black, and white adolescents differ? *Journal of Adolescent Health Care*, 11: 128-132.

Fitzpatrick, S., Johnson, J., Shragg, P., & Felice, M.E. 1987. Health care needs of Indochinese refugee teenagers. *Pediatrics*, 79: (1) 118-123 (January).

Flanagan, T.J., & Maguire, K. (Eds.), 1992. *Bureau of Justice statistics sourcebook of criminal justice statistics - 1991*. Washington, DC: United States Government Printing Office.

Flavin, D.K., & Morse, R.M. 1991. What is alcoholism?: Current definitions and diagnostic criteria and their implications for treatment. *Alcohol Health & Research World*, 15: 266-271.

Flay, B.R. 1987. Mass media and smoking cessation: A critical review. *American Journal of Public Health*, 77(2): 153-160.

Fleishman, D. 1992a. Agency mulls laboratory regulation changes: Public reaction could influence future revisions. *American Academy of Pediatrics*, 8: 1, 15.

Fleishman, D. 1992b. Study: Office labs can't handle regulatory costs. *American Academy of Pediatrics*, 8: 16, 20.

Fleishman, D. 1992c). Teens in poor community 'milk' local school clinic. *American Academy of Pediatrics*, 8: 1, 12-14, 20.

Florida Catholic Conference. 1986. *What's wrong with school-based health clinics? Questions and answers*. Tallahassee, FL: Florida Catholic Conference.

Flynn, C.C., & Harbin, G.L. 1987. Evaluating interagency coordination efforts using a multidimensional, interactional, developmental paradigm. *Remedial and Special Education*, 8: 35-44.

Ford Foundation Project on Social Welfare and the American Future. 1991. *The common good: Social welfare and the American future*. New York: Ford Foundation.

Forrest, J.D.   1990.   Adolescent reproductive behavior: An International comparison of developed countries.   In Arlene R. Stiffman and Ronald A. Feldman (Eds.), *Adolescent mental health: Research-practice annual Vol 4*, pp. 13-34. London: Jessica Kingsley Publishers.

Forste, R., & Tienda, M.   1992.   Race and ethnic variation in schooling consequences of female adolescent sexual activity. *Social Science Quarterly*, 73: 12-30.

Foster, D. 1993. The disease is adolescence. *Rolling Stone*, December 9, 1993.

Foster, S.E.   1986.   *Preventing teenage pregnancy: A public policy guide*. Washington, DC: The Council of State Policy and Planning Agencies.

Fowler, J. 1991. The Canadian experience (Viewpoint of Patrick Hewlett, MB, of Toronto). *Cortland Forum*, 4: 27.

Freimuth, V.S., Stein, J.A., & Kean, T.J.   1989.   *Searching for health information: the cancer information service model.*   Philadelphia, PA: University of Pennsylvania Press.

Friedman, E. 1991. The uninsured: From dilemma to crisis. *Journal of the American Medical Association*, 265: 2491-2495.

Friedman, H.L., & Hedlund, D.E. 1991. Counseling skills training for adolescent health: A WHO approach to meet a global need. *International Journal for the Advancement of Counselling*, 14: 59-69.

Friedman, S.B., Fisher, M., & Schonberg, S.K. (Eds.), 1992. *Comprehensive adolescent health care*. St. Louis, MO: Quality Medical Publishing, Inc.

Friedmen, S.B., & Weiner, I. 1993. Special problems of adolescents. In Robert J. Haggerty, Klaus J. Roghmann, and Ivan B. Pless (Eds.), *Child health and the community*, pp. 105-110. New Brunswick, NJ: Transaction Publishers.

Friesen, B.J., Griesbach, J., Jacobs, J. Katz-Leavy, J., & Olson, D.   1988. Improving services for families. *Children Today*, 17: 18-22.

Furstenberg, F.F, Jr. 1990. Coming of age in a changing family system. In Shirley S. Feldman, and G.R. Elliott (Eds.), *At the threshold: The developing adolescent*, pp. 147-170. Cambridge, MA: Harvard University Press.

Furstenberg, F.F., Jr. 1991. As the pendulum swings: Teenage childbearing and social concern. *Family Relations*, 40: 127-138.

Gabriel, P.H., & Hofmann, A.D. 1989. Behavioral problems. In Adele D. Greydanus and Donald E. Hofmann (Eds.), *Adolescent medicine*, pp. 553-580. Norwalk, CT: Appleton and Lange.

Galaskiewicz, J., & Shatin, D. 1981. Leadership and networking among neighborhood human service organizations. *Administrative Science Quarterly*, 26: 434-448.

Gambrell, A.E., & Kantor, L.M. 1992. The far right and fear-based abstinence-only programs. *SIECUS Report*, 21: 16-18 (December) .

Gander, M.J. & Gardiner, H.W. 1981. *Child and adolescent development.* Boston, MA: Little, Brown and Company.

Gans, J.E., Blyth, D.A., Elster, A.B., & Gaveras, L.L. 1990. *Profiles of adolescent health: America's adolescents: How Healthy are they? Volume I.* Chicago: American Medical Association.

Gans, J.E., McManus, M.A., & Newacheck, P.W. 1991. *Adolescent health : American Medical Association profiles of adolescent health care; Use, costs, and problems of access, Volume 2.* Chicago, IL: American Medical Asssociation.

Garbarino, J. 1989. Troubled youth, troubled families: The dynamics of adolescent maltreatment. In Dante Cicchetti and Vicki Carlson (Eds.), *Child maltreatment*, pp. 685-706. New York, NY: Cambridge University Press.

Gardner, S. 1989. Failure by fragmentation. *California Tomorrow*, (Fall): 26-36.

Garland, A.F., & Zigler, E. 1993. Adolescent suicide prevention: Current research and social policy implications. *American Psychologist - Special Issue on Adolescence*, 48: 169-182.

Garrison, J. 1994. Seminar summary. In Jayne Garrison, Mark D. Smith, & Douglas J. Besharov (Eds.), *Sex education in the schools*, pp. vii-xvii. Menlo Park, CA: Henry J. Kaiser Family Foundation.

Gellert, G.A., Higgins, K.V., Farley, W., & Lowery, R. 1994. Public Health and the media in california: A survey of local health Officers. *Public Health Reports*, 109(2): 284-289.

Gelles, R., & Cornell, C.P. 1990. *Intimate violence in families.* Newbury Park: Sage.

Gentry, J., & Eron, L. 1993. American Psychological Association Commission on Violence and Youth. *American Psychologist - Special Issue on Adolescence*, 48: 89.

Gerbner, G. 1985. Children's television: A national disgrace. *Pediatric Annals*, 14(12): 822-827.

Gerbner, G. 1992. Society's storyteller: How television creates the myths by which we live. *Media and Values*, 60: 8-9.

Geronimus, A.T. 1991. Teenage child bearing and social and reproductive disadvantage: The evolution of complex questions and the demise of simple answers. *Family Relations*, 40: 463-471.

Gibbs, J.T. 1988a. Health and mental health of young black males. In Jewelle Taylor Gibbs, Ann F. Brunswick, Michael E. Conner, Richard Dembo, Tom E. Larson, Rodney J. Reed, and Barbara Soloman (Eds.), *Young, black and male in America*, pp. 219-257. Dover, M.A.: Auburn House Publishing Company.

Gibbs, J.T. 1988b. The new morbidity: homicide, suicide, accidents, and life-threatening behaviors. In Jewelle T. Gibbs, Ann F. Brunswick, Michael E. Connor, Richard Dembo, Tom E. Larson, Rodney J. Reed, & Barbara Solomon. (Eds.), *Young, black, and male in America: An endangered species*, pp. 258-293. Dover, MA: Auburn House Publishing.

Gibbs, J.T., Brunswick, A.F., Conner,M.E., Dembo, R., Larson, T.E., Reed, R.J., & Soloman, B. (Eds.) 1988c. *Young, black and male In America: An endangered species*. Dover, MA: Auburn House Publishing Company.

Giblin, P.T., Poland, M.L., & Sachs, B.A. 1986. Pregnant adolescents' health-information needs. *Journal of Adolescent Health Care*, 7: 168-172.

Gilbert, G.A., Weismuller, P.C., Higgins, K.V., & Maxwell, R.M. 1992. Disclosure of AIDS in celebrities. *New England Journal of Medicine*, 327 19): 1389.

Gilchrist, L.D., Schinke, S.P., & Nurius, P. 1989. Reducing onset of habitual smoking among women. *Preventive Medicine*, 18: 235-248.

Ginsberg, C., & Loffredo, L. 1993. Violence-related attitudes and behaviors of high school students-New York City, 1992. *Journal of School Health*, 63(10): 438-440, (December).

Ginsburg, F.D. 1989. *Contested lives: The abortion debate in an American community*. Berkeley & Los Angeles, CA: University of California Press.

Ginzberg, E., & Ostow, M. 1991. Beyond universal health insurance to effective health care. *Journal of the American Medical Association*, 265: 2559-2562.

Girls Incorporated National Resource Center. 1991. Preventing adolescent pregnancy program, (unpublished brochure).

Giroux, H.A. 1987. Schooling and the politics of ethics: Beyond liberal and conservative discourses. *Journal of Education*, 169: 9-33.

Giroux, H.A. 1992. Educational leadership and the crisis of democratic government. *Educational Researcher*, 21: 4-11.

Gladstein, J., Slater Rusonis, E.J., & Heald, F.P. 1992. A comparison of inner-city and upper-middle class youths' exposure to violence. *Journal of Adolescent Health*, 13: 275-280.

Glasow, R.D. 1988. *School-based clinics, the abortion connection.* Washington, DC: National Right to Life Educational Trust Fund.

Glynn, T. 1990. School-based programs for smoking prevention. *Education Digest*, 55: 50-53.

Gold, R.B. 1990. *Abortion and women's health: A turning point for America?* New York, NY: Alan Guttmacher Institute.

Golden, O. 1991. Collaboration as a means, not an end: Serving disadvantaged families and children. In Lisbeth B. Schorr, Deborah Both, and Carol Copple (Eds.), *Effective Services for young children: Report of a workshop*, pp. 84-104. Washington, DC: National Academy Press.

Goodman, J.C. 1991. View from the forum. *Cortland Forum*, 4: 29-30, 33.

Goodwin, S. 1990. Children with special needs in england and wales: The care of hearing impairment, myelomeningocele, and adolescent pregnancy. *Pediatrics*, 1112-1116.

Goon, J.M., & Berger, D.K. 1989. A model outreach program for health care screening. *Journal of Pediatric Health Care*, 3: 305-310.

Gray, B. 1989. *Collaborating: Finding common ground for multipart problems.* San Francisco, CA: Jossey-Bass Publishers.

Green, M., & Haggerty, R.J. 1984. *Ambulatory pediatrics III.* Philadelphia: W.B. Saunders Company.

Greenberg, B.S. 1994. Content trends in media sex. In Dolf Zillman, Jennings Bryant, and Aletha C. Houston (Eds.), *Media, children and the family: Social scientific, psychodynamic and clinical perspectives,* pp. 165-180. Hillsdale, NJ: Lawrence Erlbaum Associates.

Greenstone, J.D. 1991. Culture, rationality, and the underclass. In Christopher Jencks and Paul E. Peterson (Eds.), *The urban underclass*, pp. 399-410. Washington, DC: Brookings.

Greydanus, D.E., & Hofmann, A.D. 1989a. Disorders of the skin. In Adele D. Hofmann and Donald E. Greydanus (Eds.), *Adolescent medicine*, pp. 279-306. Norwalk, CT: Appleton and Lange.

Greydanus, D.E., & Hofmann, A.D. 1989b. Eyes, ears, nose, mouth, and throat. In Adele D. Hofmann and Donald E. Greydanus (Eds.), *Adolescent medicine*, pp. 45-67. Norwalk, CT: Appleton and Lange.

Greydanus, D.E., & Hofmann, A.D. 1989c). Infectious disease. In Adele D. Hofmann and Donald E. Greydanus (Eds.), *Adolescent medicine*, pp. 307-325. Norwalk, CT: Appleton and Lange.

Grochowski, E.C., & Bach, S. 1994. The ethics of decision making with adolescents: What a physician ought to know. In Donald E. Greydanus, Kimball A. Miller, and Helen D. Pratt (Eds.). *Adolescent medicine: Frontiers of academic medicine and health care delivery in the 1900s,* 5 (3): 485-495. Philadelphia, PA: Hanley & Belfus, Inc.

Gross, J. 1994. Sex educators for young see new virtue in chastity. In Jayne Garrison, Mark D. Smith, & Douglas J. Besharov (Eds.), *Sex education in the schools*, pp. 75-81. Menlo Park, CA: Henry J. Kaiser Family Foundation.

Grumbach, K. 1991. Liberal benefits, conservative spending: The physicians for a national health program proposal. *Journal of the American Medical Association*, 265: 2549-2554.

Guetzloe, E. 1988. What are the schools responsibilities?: School prevention of suicide, violence, and abuse. *Educational Digest*, 54: 46-49.

Guidubaldi, J., & Cleminshaw, H. 1985. Divorce, family health, and child adjustment. *Family Relations*, 34: 35-41.

Gullotta, J.P., Adams, G.R., & Mayor, R.M. (Eds.). 1993. *Adolescent sexuality*. Newbury Park, CA: Sage Publications.

Hackstaff, K.B. 1994. *Divorce culture: A breach in gender relations.* Doctoral Dissertation, Department of Sociology, University of California, Berkeley, CA.

Haggerty, R.J., & Roghmann, K.J. (Eds.). 1993. *Child health and the community.* New Brunswick, NJ: Transaction Publishers.

Haggerty, R.J., Roghmann, K.J., & Pless, I.B. 1993. Summary and implications: Where do we stand? In Robert J. Haggerty, Klaus J. Roghmann, and Ivan B. Pless (Eds.), *Child health and the community,* pp. 312-331. New Brunswick, NJ: Transaction Publishers.

Hale, J.P. 1988. The bishops blunder. *America,* 158: 156-158, 171.

Ham, M., & Larson , R. 1993. Stress and 'storm and stress' in early adolescence: The relationship of negative events with dysphoric affect. *Developmental Psychology,* 29: 130-140.

Hamburg, B.A. 1989. Adolescent health care and disease prevention in the Americas. In David Hamburg and Norman Sartorius (Eds.), *Health and behavior: Selected perspectives,* pp. 127-147. New York, NY: Cambridge University Press.

Hamburg, D.A. 1992. *Today's children.* New York, NY: Times Books.

Hamburg, D.A. & Sartorius, N. 1989. *Health and behavior: Selected perspectives.* New York, NY: Cambridge University Press.

Hammond, W.R., & Yeng, B. 1993. Psychologist role in the public health response to assaultive violence among young African-American men. *American Psychologist - Special Issue on Adolescence,* 48: 142-154.

Hanagan, T.J., & Maguire, K. (Eds.). 1992. *Bureau of Justice statistics sourcebook of criminal justice statistics - 1991.* Washington, DC: United States Government Printing Office.

Handler, A. 1990. The correlates of the initiation of sexual intercourse among young urban black females. *Journal of Youth and Adolescence,* 19: 159-171.

Hansen, W. 1993. School-based alcohol prevention programs. *Alcohol Health & Research World,* pp. 54-58.

Hanson, J.G., Crase, S.J., & Stockdale, D.F. 1993. Maternal attitudes of pregnant and/or parenting, and nonpregnant, nonparenting adolescents. Paper presented at the National Conference on Family Relationa, 55th Annual Conference, Baltimore, MD.

Harbin, G.L., & McNulty, B. 1990. Policy implementation: perspectives on service coordination and interagency cooperation. In Samuel J. Musels and Jack P. Shonkoff (Eds.), *Handbook of early childhood intervention*, pp. 700-721. New York, NY: Cambridge University Press.

Hardy, J.B. 1988. Teenage pregnancy: An American dilemma. In Helen Wallace, George Ryan, and Allan C. Oglesby (Eds.), *Maternal and child health practices*, pp. 539-554. Oakland, CA: Third Party Publishing Company.

Hardy, J.B. 1991. *Adolescent pregnancy in an urban environment: Issues, programs, and evaluation.* Janet B. Hardy and Laurie Schwab Zabin (Eds.). Washington, DC: Urban Institute Press.

Harkness, S., Super, C.M., & Keefer, C.H. 1992. Culture and ethnicity. In Melvin D. Levine, William B. Carey, and Allen C. Crocker (Eds.), *Developmental-behavioral pediatrics*, pp. 103-108. Philadelphia, PA: W.B.Saunders Company.

Harrington, C. 1991. A national long term care program for the United States. *Journal of the American Medical Association*, 266: 3023-3029.

Harrington, D. 1995. Family violence and development during adolescence. In Katherine Kaufer Christoffel & Carol W. Runyan (Eds.), *Adolescent medicine: adolescent injuries: Epidemiology and prevention*, 6 (2): 199-206. Philadelphia, PA: Hanley & Belfus, Inc.

Hauser, S.T., Jacobson, A.M., Wertlieb, D. Brink, S., & Wentworth, S. 1985. The contribution of family environment to perceived competence and illness adjustment in diabetic and acutely ill adolescents. *Family Relations*, 34: 99-108.

Hayes, C.D. 1987. *Risking the future: Adolescent sexuality, pregnancy, and childbearing.* Washington, DC: National Academy Press.

Hayes, C.D. 1991. *Beyond rhetoric: A new American agenda for children and families.* Washington, DC: National Commission on Children.

Heaton, C.J., & Smith, M.A. 1989. The diaphragm. *American Family Physician*, 39(5): 231-236.

Hechinger, F.M. 1992. *Fateful choices: Healthy youth for the 21st century.* New York, NY:Hill and Wang.

Hendee, W.R. (Ed.) 1991. *The health of adolescents.* San Francisco, CA: Jossey-Bass Publishers.

Hendren, R.L., & Strasburger, V.C. 1993. Rock music and music videos. In Victor C. Strasburger and George A. Comstock (Eds.). *Adolescent medicine: Adolescents and the media,* 4 (3): 577-588. Philadelphia: Hanley & Belfus, Inc.

Henriot, P.J., DeBerri, E.P., & Schultheis, M.J. 1988. *Catholic social teaching: Our best kept secret.* Washington, DC: Center of Concern.

Henry, C.S., Stephenson, A.L., Hanson, M.F., & Hargett, W. 1993. Adolescent suicide and families: An ecological approach. *Adolescence,* 28: 291-308.

Henshaw, S.K. 1990. Induced abortions: A world review, 1990. *Family Planning Perspectives,* 22 (2): 76-89.

Henshaw, S.K. 1992. Induced abortion: A world view. In J. Douglas Butler and David F. Walbert (Eds). *Abortion, medicine, and the law,* pp. 406-436. New York: Facts On File.

Henshaw, S.K. 1993. Teenage abortion, birth and pregnancy statistics by state, 1988. *Family Planning Perspectives,* 25: 122-126.

Henshaw, S.K. 1994. Abortion services under national health insurance: The examples of england and france. *Family Planning Perspectives,* 26: 87-89.

Henshaw, S.K., & Van Vort, J. 1994. Abortion services in the United States, 1991 and 1992. Family Planning Perspectives, 26: 100-106 & 112.

Hensly, W.R. (Ed.). 1990. *Stedman's medical dictionary.* Baltimore, MD: Williams and Wilkins.

Hepworth, J., & Jackson, M. 1985. Health care for families: Models of collaboration between family therapists and family physicians. *Family Relations,* 34: 123-127.

Herceg-Baron, R., Harris, K.M., Armstrong, K. Furstenberg, F., & Shea, J. 1990. Factors differentiating effective use of contraception among adolescents. In Arlene R. Stiffman and Ronald A. Feldman (Eds.), *Adolescent mental health: Research-practice annual Vol. 4,* pp. 37-50. London: Jessica Kingsley Publishers.

Hibbard, R.A., Ingersoll, G. M., & Orr, D.P. 1990. Behavioral risk, emotional risk, and child abuse among adolescents in a nonclinical setting. *Pediatrics*, 86: 896-901.

Hibbard, R.A., Spence, C., Tzeng, O.C.S., Zollinger, T., & Orr, D.P. 1992. Child abuse and mental health among adolescents in dependent care. *Journal of Adolescent Health*, 13: 121-127.

Hilfiker, D. 1994. *Not all of us are saints: A doctor's journey with the poor.* New York, NY: Hill and Wang.

Himes, K., & Himes, M. 1993. *Fullness of faith: The public significance of theology.* New York, NY: Paulist.

Hodgman, C. 1989. Depression, suicide, out-of-control reactions and psychoses. In Arlene D. Hofmann & Donald E. Greydanus (Eds.), *Adolescent medicine*, pp. 581-591. Norwalk, CT: Appleton and Lange.

Hodgman, C. 1990. Adolescent depression and suicide. In Victor C. Strasburger and Donald E. Greydanus (Eds.), *Adolescent medicine: The at-risk adolescent*, 1 (1): 81-95. Philadelphia, PA: Hanley & Belfus, Inc.

Hofferth, S.L., & Hayes, C.D., 1987. *Risking the future, Volume II.* Washington, DC: National Academy Press.

Holahan, J. 1991. An American approach to health system reform. *Journal of the American Medical Association*, 265: 2537-2540.

Hollander, D. 1993. Some teenagers say they might not seek health care if they could not be assured of confidentiality. *Family Planning Perspectives*, 25(4.

Holund, U. 1990. Promoting change of adolescents' sugar consumption: The "learning by teaching" study. *Health Education Research*, 5: 451-458.

Horwitz, E.L. 1991. World here we come. *American Association of University Women*, 14-19.

Howard, M. 1985. Postponing sexual involvement among adolescents. *Journal of Adolescent Health Care*, 6: 271-277.

Howard, M. 1992. Delaying the start of intercourse among adolescents. *Adolescent medicine: Adolescent sexuality: Preventing unhealthy consequences*, 3: 181-193. Philadelphia, PA: Hanley & Belfus, Inc.

Howard, M., & McCabe, J. 1990. Helping teenagers postpone sexual involvement. *Family Planning Perspectives*, 22: 21.

Howard, M., & McCabe, J. 1992. An information and skills approach for younger teens: Postponing sexual involvement program. In Brent C. Miller, Josefina J. Card, Roberta L. Paikoff, & James L. Peterson (Eds.), *Preventing Adolescent Pregnancy*, pp. 83-109. Newbury Park, CA: Sage Publications.

Hsiao, V. 1986. Relationship between urinary tract infection and contraceptive methods. *Society for Adolescent Medicine.* New York, NY: Elsevier Science Publishing Co., Inc.

Huang, L.N., & Gibbs, J.T. 1990. Future directions: Implications for research, training, and practice. In Jewelle Taylor Gibbs, Larke Nahme Huang, and associates (Eds.), *Children of color: Psychological interventions with minority youth*, pp. 375-403. San Francisco, CA: Jossey Bass Publishers.

Huffman, H.A. 1993. Character education without turmoil. *Educational Leadership*, 51: 24-26.

Hutchins, V.L., & McPherson, M. 1991. National agenda for children with special health needs: Social policy for the 1990s through the 21st century. *American Psychologist*, 46: 141-143.

Hutchinson, G.E., Freedson, P.S., Ward, A. & Rippe, J. 1990. Ideal to real - implementing a youth fitness program. *Journal of Physical Education, Recreation, and Dance*, 61: 52-58.

Igra, V., & Millstein, S.G. 1993. Current status and approaches to improving preventive services for adolescents. *Journal of the American Medical Association*, 269: 1408-1412.

Inclan, J.E., & Herron, D.G. 1990. Puerto Rican adolescents. In Jewelle Taylor Gibbs, Larke Nahme Huang, and associates (Eds.), *Children of color: Psychological interventions with minority youth*, pp. 251-277. San Francisco, CA: Jossey-Bass Publishers.

Ingraham, G.C., & Miller, N. 1993. Attitudes, behavior, and HIV: Are we preparing our children? *NASSP Bulletin*, 77: 16-20.

Institute of Medicine. 1989. *Research on children and adolescents with mental, behavioral, and developmental disorders: Mobilizing a national initiative.* Washington, DC: National Academy Press.

Irwin, C.E. 1990. The theoretical concept of at-risk adolescents. In Victor C. Strasburger and Donald E. Greydanus (Eds.), *Adolescent medicine: The at-risk adolescent,* 1 (1): 1-14. Philadelphia, PA: Hanley & Belfus, Inc.

Jack, J. 1991. The Canadian experience (Viewpoint of Patrick Hewlett, MB, of Toronto). Cortland *Forum,* 4: 27.

Jenkins, E., & Bell, C. 1992. Adolescent violence: Can it be cured? *Adolescent medicine: Psychosocial issues in adolescents,* 3: 71-86. Philadelphia, PA: Hanley & Belfus, Inc.

Jessor, R. 1993. Successful adolescent development among youth in high risk settings. *America Psychologist - Special Issue on Adolescence,* 48: 117-126.

Joffe, A., Radius, S., & Gall, M. 1988. Health counseling for adolescents. What they want, what they get, who gives it. *Pediatrics,* 82: 481-485.

John Paul II, Pope. 1980. Address to the Confederation of Family Advisory Bureaus of Christian Inspiration. *Insegnamenti III,* 2: 1453-1454.

John Paul II, Pope. 1981. *Familiaris consortio.* Washington, DC: Office of Publishing Services, United States Catholic Conference.

John Paul II, Pope. 1987. *Sollicitudo rei socialis.* Boston, MA: St. Paul Books and Media.

John Paul II, Pope. 1989. *Christifdeles laici.* Boston, MA: Daughters of St. Paul.

John Paul II, Pope. 1991. *Centesimus annus.* Washington, DC: Office of Publishing Services, United States Catholic Conference.

John Paul II, Pope, & the USCC Administrative Board. 1987. The many faces of AIDS: A gospel response. *Origins NC Documentary Service,* 17: #28 481-496.

Johnson, C.M. 1992. *Vanishing dreams: The economic plight of America's young families.* Washington, DC: The Children's Defense Fund.

Johnson, H.W., McLaughlin, J.A., & Christensen, M. 1982. Interagency collaboration: Driving and restraining forces. *Exceptional Children,* 48: 395-399.

Johnson, K., & Moore, A. 1990. *Improving health programs for low-income youths: Adolescent pregnancy prevention clearinghouse.* Washington, DC: Children's Defense Fund.

Johnson, L., O'Malley, P.M., & Bachman, J.G. 1991. *Drug use among American high school seniors, college students and young adults, 1975-1990.* Rockville, MD: U.S. Department of Health and Human Services, Public Health Service, Alcohol, Drug Abuse, and Mental Health Administration, National Institute on Drug Abuse.

Johnson, R.L. 1989. Adolescent growth and development. In Adele D. Greydanus and Donald E.Hofmann (Eds.) *Adolescent medicine*, pp. 9-15. Norwalk, CT: Appleton and Lange.

Johnson-Powell, G. 1992. Poverty. In Stanford B. Friedman, Martin Fisher, and S. Kenneth Schonberg (Eds.), *Comprehensive adolescent health care*, pp. 692-698. St. Louis, MO: Quality Medical Publishing, Inc.

Jones, J.E. 1985. Fertility-related care. In Harriette McAdoo and T.M. Jim Parham (Eds.), *Services to young families.* Washington, DC: American Public Welfare Association.

Jorgensen, S.R. 1991. Project taking charge: An evaluation of an adolescent pregnancy prevention program. *Family Relations*, 40: 373-380.

Jorgensen, S.R., Potts, V., & Camp, B. 1993. Project taking charge: Six-month follow-up of a pregnancy prevention program for early adolescents. *Family Relations*, 42: 401-406.

Joseph P. Kennedy, Jr. Foundation. 1982. *A community of caring.* New York, NY: Walker Publishing.

Jurich, J.A., Rupp, M., Lansinger, T., & Erler, C. 1993. Factors associated with high-risk sexual behavior in college students. Unpublished paper, West Lafayette, IN: Purdue University.

Kachur, S.P., Potter, L.B., Powell, K.E., & Rosenberg, M.L. 1995. Suicide: Epidemiology, prevention, and treatment. In Katherine Kaufer Christoffel & Carol W. Runyan (Eds.), *Adolescent medicine: Adolescent injuries: Epidemiology and prevention*, 6 (2): 183-198. Philadelphia, PA: Hanley & Belfus, Inc.

Kagan, S.L. 1991. *United we stand: Collaboration for child care and early education services.* New York, NY: Teachers College Press.

Kahn, A.J., & Kamerman, S.B. 1980. *Social services in international perspective: The emergence of the sixth system.* New Brunswick, NJ: Transaction Books.

Kahn, A.J., & Kamerman, S.B. 1992. *Integrating services integration: An overview of initiatives, issues, and possibilities.* New York, NY: National Center for Children in Poverty.

Kamarck, E.C., & Galston, W.A. 1990. *Putting children first: A progressive family policy for the 1990's.* Washington, DC: Progressive Policy Institute.

Kamerow, D.B., Pincus, H.A., & Macdonald, D.I. 1986. Alcohol abuse, other drug abuse and mental disorders in medical practice: Prevalence, costs, recognition and treatment. *Journal of the American Medical Association,* 255: 2054-2057.

Kani, J., & Adler, M.W. 1992. Epidemiology of pelvic inflammatory disease. In Gary S. Berger and Lars V. Westrom (Eds.), *Pelvic inflammatory disease,* pp. 7-23. New York, NY: Raven Press Ltd.

Kansas Employer Coalition on Health, Task Force on Long-Term Solutions, The. 1991. A framework for reform of the us health care financing and provision system. *Journal of the American Medical Association,* 265: 2529-2531.

Kaplan, A.S., & Woodside, D.B. 1987. Biological aspects of anorexia nervosa and bulimia nervosa. *Journal of Consulting and Clinical Psychology,* 55: 645-653.

Kaplan, A.S. 1990. Biomedical variables in the eating disorders. *Canadian Journal of Psychiatry,* 35: 745-753.

Kaplan, M.E., & Friedman, S.B. 1994. Reciprocal influences between chronic illness and adolescent development. In Robert T. Brown and Susan M. Coupey (Eds.), *Adolescent medicine: Chronic and disabling disorders,* 5 (2): 211-222. Philadelphia, PA: Hanley & Belfus, Inc.

Kassberg, M., & David, J. 1991. OBG care for teens: Cooperation is the key. *Pediatric Management,* 4: 39-46.

Kazdin, A. 1993. Adolescent mental health. *American Psychologist - Special Issue on Adolescence,* 48: 127-141.

Kelleher, K. 1991. Free clinics: A solution that can work. . . now! *Journal of the American MedicalAssociation,* 266: 838-840.

Kenney, R. 1989. A guide to sexual abstinence counseling. *Contemporary Pediatrics,* 6: 83-84, 87-88, 91-92, 95.

Ketterlinus, R.D., Lamb, M., & Nitz, K. 1991. Developmental and ecological sources of stress among adolescent parents. *Family Relations,* 40: 435-441.

Kiesler, C.A. 1991. Homelessness and public policy priorities. *American Psychologist*, 46: 1245-1252.

Kilbourne, B.W., Buehler, J.W., & Rogers, M.J. 1990. AIDS as a cause of death in children, adolescents, and young adults. *American Journal of Public Health*, 80: 499-500.

Kilbourne, J. 1993. Killing us softly: Gender roles in advertising. In Victor C. Strasburger and George A. Comstock, *Adolescent medicine: Adolescents and the media*, 4 (3): 635-650. Philadelphia: Hanley & Belfus, Inc.

Kinard, E.M. 1990. Children of adolescents: Behavioral and emotional functioning. In Arlene R. Stiffman and Ronald A. Feldman (Eds.), *Adolescent mental health: A research-practice annual*, pp. 239-262. London: Jessica Kingsley Publishers.

Kinast, R.L. 1985. *Caring for society: A theological interpretation of lay ministry.* Chicago, IL: T. More Press.

Kinast, R.L. 1990. Health care ministry: A handbook for chaplains. In Helen Hayes and Cornelius J. Van der Poel (Eds.), *Caring for God's Covenant of Freedom: A theology of pastoral care*, pp. 7-21. Mahwah, NJ: Paulist.

King, C.T., *Strategies for resolving eligibility conflicts and promoting program coordination.* Unpublished Paper, University of Texas.

King, P. (Ed.), 1994. *Catholic women and abortion: Stories of healing.* Kansas City, MO: Sheed & Ward.

Kipke, M.D., & Hein, K. 1990. Acquired Immunodeficiency Syndrome (AIDS) in adolescents. In Manuel Schydlower and Mary-Ann Shafer (Eds.), *Adolescent medicine: AIDS and other sexually transmitted diseases*, 1 (3): 429-449. Philadelphia, PA: Hanley & Belfus, Inc.

Kirby, D. 1988. Sexuality education. In Helen M. Wallace, George Ryan, and Allan C. Oglesby (Eds.), *Maternal and child health practices*, pp. 555-562. Oakland, CA: Third Party Publishing Company.

Kirby, D. 1992. School-based programs to reduce sexual risk-taking behaviors. *Journal of School Health*, 62: 280-287.

Kirby, D. 1994. Sexuality and HIV education programs in schools. In Jayne Garrison, Mark D. Smith, & Douglas J. Besharov (Eds.), *Sex education in the schools*, pp. 1-41. Menlo Park, CA: Henry J. Kaiser Family Foundation.

Kirby, D., Waszak, C.S., & Ziegler, J. 1989. *An assessment of six school-based clinics: services, impact and potential.* Washington, DC: Center for Population Options.

Kirkendall, L.A. 1982. Commentary on Shornack's article. *Family Relations,* 31: 545.

Kirkman, L. 1991. Health insurance values and implementation in the Netherlands and the Federal Republic of Germany: An alternative path to universal coverage. *Journal of the American Medical Association,* 265: 2496-2502.

Kisker, E.E. 1985. Teenagers talk about sex, pregnancy and contraception. *Family Planning Perspectives,* 17: 83-90.

Kittrie, N.N. 1971. *The right to be different: Deviance and enforced therapy.* Baltimore, MD: John Hopkins University Press.

Klein, J.D., Brown, J.D., Childers, K.W., Oliveri, J., Porter, C., & Dykers, C. 1992. Adolescents' risky behavior and mass media use. *Pediatrics,* 82: 24-31.

Klein, J.D., Starnes, S.A., Kotelchuck, M. Earp, J.A., DeFriese, G.H., & Loda, F.A. 1992. *Comprehensive adolescent health services in the United States.* Chapel Hill, NC: Center for Health Promotion and Disease Prevention.

Klitsch, M. 1994a. Abortion funding cutoff will likely cost Michigan far more than it saves. *Family Planning Perspectives,* 26: 92-93.

Klitsch, M. 1994b. Risky youth in inner cities. *Family Planning Perspectives,* 25: 194.

Klitsch, M. 1994c). Sex and the moving teen. *Family Planning Perspectives,* 26: 98-99.

Klitsch, M. 1994d). Unwanted sex among the young. *Family Planning Perspectives,* :50.

Knitzer, J. 1982. *The failure of public responsibility to children and adolescents in need of mental health services: Unclaimed children.* Washington, DC: Children's Defense Fund.

Knitzer, J. 1984. Mental health services to children and adolescents: A national view of public policies. *American Psychologist,* 39: 905-911.

Koonin, L.M., Kochanek, K.D., Smith, J.C., & Ramick, M. 1992. Abortion surveillance, United States, 1988. In J. Douglas Butler and David F. Walbert (Eds.), *Abortion, medicine, and the law*, pp. 458-481. New York, NY: Facts On File.

Koonin, L.M., Smith, J.C., Ramick, M., & Lawson, H.W. 1992. Abortion surveillance--United States, 1989. *Morbidity and Mortality Weekly Report*, 41: 1-33.

Koop, C.E. 1992. The U.S. Surgeon General's report on the health effects of abortion. In J. Douglas Butler and David F. Walbert (Eds.), *Abortion, medicine, and the law*, pp. 731-744. New York, NY: Facts on File.

Koteskey, R.L. 1991. Adolescence as a cultural invention. In Donald Radcliff and James A. Davies (Eds.), *Handbook of youth ministry*, pp. 42-69. Birmingham, AL: R.E.P. Books.

Kovacs, M. 1989. Affective disorders in children and adolescents. *American Psychology*, 44: 209-215.

Kovar, M.G., & Dawson , D. 1988. Health of adolescents. In Helen M. Wallace, George Ryan, and Allan C. Oglesby (Eds.), *Maternal and child health practices*, pp. 521-530. Oakland, CA: Third Party Publishing Company.

Kraus, J.F., & Conroy, C. 1984. Mortality and morbidity from injuries in sports and recreation. *Annual Review of Public Health*, 5: 163-192.

Kraus, W.A. 1980. *Collaboration in organizations: Alternatives to hierarchy.* New York, NY: Human Sciences Press, Inc.

Kreipe, R.E., & Sahler, O.J. 1991. Physical growth and development in normal adolescents. In William R. Hendee (Ed.), *The health of adolescents*, pp. 21-57. San Francisco, CA: Jossey-Bass Publishing Company.

Kronick, R. 1989. *Adolescent health insurance status: Analyses of trends in coverage and preliminary estimates of the effects of an employer mandate and medicaid expansion on the uninsured.* Washington, DC: U.S. Government Printing Office.

Ku, L., Sonenstein, F., & Pleck, J. 1992. The Association of AIDS Education and Sex Education With Sexual Behavior and Condom Use Among Teenage Men. *Family Planning Perspectives*, 24: 100-106.

Kulig, J. 1996. Gonococcal infection in the adolescent male. In Paul G. Dyment (Ed.), *Adolescent medicine: Male reproductive health,* 7 (1): 83-92. Philadelphia, PA: Hanley & Belfus, Inc.

La Fromboise, T.D., & Low, K.G. 1990. American Indian children and adolescents. In Jewelle Taylor Gibbs, Larke Nahne Huang, and Associates (Eds.), *Children of color: Psychological interventions with minority youth.* San Francisco, CA: Jossey-Bass Publishers.

Lamarine, R. 1989. The dilemma of Native American health. *Health Education,* 20: 15-18.

Land, H. 1987. Children having children. *Society,* 24: 36-40.

Land, P.S. 1988. *Shaping welfare consensus: U.S. Catholic Bishops contributions.* Washington, DC: Center of Concern.

Langwell, K., & Menke, T. 1991. *Rising health care costs: Causes, implications, and strategies.* Washington, DC: U.S. Government Printing Office.

Larsson, E.V., & Christian, W.P. 1992. Legal issues. In Melvin D. Levine, William B. Carey, and Allen C. Crocker (Eds.), *Developmental-behavioral pediatrics,* pp. 771-781. Philadelphia, PA: W.B.Saunders Company.

Lavin, A.T., Shapiro, G.R., & Weill, K.S. 1992. Creating an agenda for school-based health promotion: A review of 25 selected reports. *Journal of School Health,* 62: 212-228.

Lear, J.G. 1992. School-based health care. In Stanford B. Friedman, Martin Fisher, and S. Kenneth Schonberg (Eds.), *Comprehensive adolescent health care,* pp. 899-902. St. Louis, MO: Quality Medical Publishing, Inc.

Lear, J.G., Foster, H.W., & Baratz, J.A. 1989. The high-risk young people's program. *Journal of Adolescent Health Care,* 10: 224-230.

Lear, J.G., Gleicher, H.B., St. Germaine, A., & Porter, P.J. 1991. Reorganizing health care for adolescents: The experience of school-based adolescent health care program. *Journal of Adolescent Health,* 12: 450-455.

Leary, W.E. 1989. Campus AIDS survey finds Threat is real but not yet rampant. *New York Times,* May 23, Section C: 12.

LeBeau, J. 1988. The "silver-spoon" syndrome in the super rich: The pathologic linkage of affluence and narcissism in family systems. *American Journal of Psychotherapy,* XLII (3): 425-436.

Leming, J.S. 1993. In search of effective character education. *Educational Leadership*, 51: 63-71.

Leo XIII, Pope. 1939. *Rerum novarum*. New York, NY: The Paulist Press.

Levenson, P.M., Morrow, J.R., Morgan, W.C., & Pfefferbaum, B.J. 1986. Health information sources and preferences as perceived by adolescents, pediatricians, teachers and school nurses. *Journal of Early Adolescence*, 6: 183-195.

Levenson, P.M., Pfefferbaum, B., & Morrow, J.R. 1987. Disparities in adolescent-physician views of teen health information concerns. *Journal of Adolescent Health Care*, 8: 171-176.

Levenson, P.M., Smith, P.B., & Morrow, J.R. 1986. A comparison of physician-patient views of teen prenatal information needs. *Journal of Adolescent Health Care*, 7: 6-11.

Levine, M.D. 1989. Attention and memory: Progression and Variation during the elementary school years. *Pediatric Annals*, 18: 366-372.

Levitan, S.A., Mangum, G.L., & Pines, M.W. 1989. *A proper inheritance: Investing in the self-sufficiency of poor families*. Washington, DC: The George Washington University.

Levy, A., & Merry, U. 1986. *Organizational transformation*. New York, NY: Praeger Publishers.

Lewinsohn, P.M., Rohde, P., & Seeley, J.R. 1994. Psychosocial risk factors for future adolescent suicide attempts. *Journal of Consulting and Clinical Psychology*, 62: 297-305.

Li, G., Baker, S.P., & Frattaroli, S. 1995. Epidemiology and prevention of traffic-related injuries among adolescents. In Katherine Kaufer Christoffel & Carol W. Runyan (Eds.), *Adolescent medicine: Adolescent injuries: Epidemiology and prevention*, 6 (2): 135-152. Philadelphia, PA: Hanley & Belfus, Inc.

Lickona, T. 1993a. The return of character education. *Educational Leadership*, 51: 6-11.

Lickona, T. 1993b. Where sex education went wrong. *Educational Leadership*, 51: 84-89.

Lidegaard, O., & Helm, P. 1990. Pelvic inflammatory disease: The influence of contraceptive, sexual, and social life events. *Contraception*, 41: 475-483.

Lieu, T.A., Newacheck, P.W., & McManus, M.A. 1993. Race, ethnicity, and access to ambulatory care among US adolescents. *American Journal of Public Health*, 83: 960-965.

Lin, W.T., & Yu, E.S.H. 1985. Ethnicity, mental health, and the urban delivery system. In Lionel Moldanado and Joan Moore, (Eds.), *urban ethnicity in the United States: New immigrants and old minorities*, pp. 211-247. Beverly Hills, CA: Sage Publishing

Lippitt, R., & Van Til, J. 1981. Can we achieve a collaborative community? Issues, imperatives, potential. *Journal of Voluntary Action Research*, 10: 7-17.

Lipsitz, J. 1980. *Growing up forgotten.* New Brunswick, NJ: Transaction Publishers.

Litt, I.F. 1983. Menstrual problems during adolescence. *Pediatrics in Review*, 4: 203-212.

Litt, I.F. 1987. Special health problems during adolescence. In Richard E. Behrman, Victor C. Vaughan, and Waldo E. Nelson (Eds.), *Nelson textbook of pediatrics*, pp. 436-454. Philadelphia, PA: W.B. Saunders.

Liu, J.T., & Rosenbaum, S. 1992. *Medicaid and childhood immunizations: A national study.* Washington, DC: Children's Defense Fund.

Liu, W.T., & Yu, E.S.H. 1985. Ethnicity, mental health, and the urban delivery system. In Lionel Moldonado, and Joan Moore (Eds.), *Urban ethnicity in the United States: New immigrants and old minorities*, pp. 211-247. Beverly Hills, CA: Sage.

Lockwood, A.L. 1993. A Letter to character educators. *Educational Leadership*, 51: 72-75.

Long, K.A. 1985. Pitfalls to avoid and positive approaches in the nurse-adolescent relationship. *Perspectives in Psychiatric Care*, 23: 22-26.

Lovato, C.Y., Allensworth, D.D., & Chan, M. 1989. *School health in America: An assessment of state policies to protect and improve the health of students.* Kent, OH: American School Health Association.

Lovett, J., & Wald, M.S. 1985. Physician attitudes toward confidential care for adolescents. *The Journal of Pediatrics*, 106: 517-521.

Luder, E. 1992. Cultural aspects of nutrition in adolescents. In Michael P. Nussbaum and Johanna T. Dwyer (Eds.), *Adolescent medicine: Adolescent nutrition and eating disorder*, 3 (3): 405-416. Philadelphia, PA: Hanley & Belfus, Inc.

Luker, K. 1984. *Abortion and the politics of motherhood.* Los Angeles, CA: University of California Press.

Lundberg, G.D. 1991. National health care reform: An aura of inevitability is upon us. *Journal of the American Medical Association*, 265: 2566-2567.

Luongo, P. 1992. Steps and strategies at the county level: The Montgomery County experience in Maryland. In Wendy Snyder and Theodore Ooms (Eds.), *Empowering families, helping adolescents: Family-centered treatment of adolescents with alcohol drug abuse and mental health problems*, pp. 157-168. Washington, DC: United States Government Printing Office.

Lynch, T., & Preister, S. 1988. *A Family perspective in church and society.* Washington, DC: U.S. Catholic Conference.

MacDonald, D.I. 1988a. The problem. *Adolescent Wellness Newsletter*, 1. Lyndhurst, NJ: Health Learning Systems Inc.

MacDonald, D.I. 1988b. Substance abuse. In Helen Wallace, George Ryan, and Allan C. Oglesby (Eds.), *Maternal and child health practices*, pp. 573-581. Oakland, CA: Third Party Publishing Company.

Macionis, J.J. 1995. *Sociology.* Englewood Cliffs, NJ: Prentice Hall.

Maher, L.T. 1986. *Memoranda to pastors and parishioners regarding health clinics in public schools.* Diocese of San Diego: Unpublished memo, from Office For Apostolic Ministry.

Males, M. 1992. Use of a school referendum to deter teen-age tobacco use. *Journal of School Health*, 62: 229-232.

Males, M. 1993a. School-age pregnancy: Why hasn't prevention worked? *Journal of School Health*, 63 (10): 429-432.

Males, M. 1993b. Schools, society, and 'teen' pregnancy. *Phi Delta Kappan*, 74: 566-568.

Malinowski, M.J. 1992. Hello, Dad. This is your daughter. Can I get an abortion?: An essay on the minor's right to a confidential abortion. In J. Douglas Butler and David F. Walbert (Eds.), *Abortion, medicine, and the law*, pp. 182-222. New York: Facts on File.

Mannion, M.T. 1992. *Abortion and healing: A cry to be whole.* Kansas City, MO: Sheed & Ward.

Mannion, M. T. (Ed.) 1994. *Post-abortion aftermath: A comprehensive consideration.* Kansas City, MO: Sheed & Ward.

Marks, A., & Fisher, M. 1987. Health assessment and screening during adolescence. *Pediatrics*, 80: 135-158.

Martin, T.M. 1990. *The challenge of Christian marriage: Marriage in scripture, history, and contemporary life.* New York, NY: Paulist Press.

Martinson, M.C. 1982. Interagency services: A new era for an old idea. *Exceptional Children*, 48: 389-394.

Maschhof, T.A., Chandler, N.S., Armstrong, S. & Hansen, R. 1981. The media as an approach to adolescent health education. *Journal of Adolescent Health Care*, 1: 221-224.

Mattessich, P.W., & Monsey, B.R. 1992. *Collaboration: What makes it work - A review of research literature on factors influencing successful collaboration.* St. Paul, MN: Amherst H. Wilder Foundation.

McAnarney, E. 1993. Home alone: Potential implications for adolescents. *Pediatrics*, 92(1): 146-148.

McCarthy, P. 1992. Steps and strategies at the state level: The Delaware experience. In Wendy Snyder and Theodora Ooms (Eds.), *Empowering families, helping adolescents: Family-centered treatment of adolescents with alcohol drug abuse, and mental health problems*, pp. 145-156. Washington, DC: United States Government Printing Office.

McCormick, R.A. 1984. *Health and medicine in the Catholic tradition: Tradition in transition.* New York, NY: Crossroad.

McCormick, R.A. 1988. AIDS: The shape of the ethical challenge. *America*, 158: 147-152, 154.

McCubbin, H.I., Needle, R.H., & Wilson, M. 1985. Adolescent health risk behaviors: Family stress and adolescent coping as critical factors. *Family Relations*, 34: 51-62.

McGeady, M.R. 1991. Disconnected kids: An American tragedy. *America*, 164: 639-645.

McGinnis, J.M. 1987. Introduction to the National Children and Youth Fitness Study II. *Journal of Physical Education, Recreation, and Dance*, 58: 50.

McGuire, A. 1989. Fires, Cigarettes, and Advocacy. *Law, Medicine, and Health Care*, 17: 73-77.

McKee, M. 1992. Studies show businesses over pay for health care. *American Academy of Pediatrics*, 8: 5.

McLain, L.G., & Reynolds, S. 1989. Sports injuries in a high school. *Pediatrics*, 84: 446-450.

McManus, M., McCarthy, E., Kozak, L.J., & Newacheck, P. 1991. Hospital use by adolescents and young adults. *Journal of Adolescent Health*, 12: 107-115.

McManus, M.A., & Newacheck, P.W. 1989. Rural maternal, child, and adolescent health. *Health Services Research*, 23: 807-848.

McShane, D. 1988. Analysis of mental health research with American Indian youth. *Journal of Adolescence*, 11: 87-116.

McWhinney, I.R., & Patterson, J.M. 1992. In Russell J. Sawa (Ed.), *Family theory in family medicine*, pp. 40-49. Newbury Park, CA: Sage Publications.

Melaville, A.I., & Blank, M.J. 1991. *What it takes: Structuring interagency partnerships to connect children and families with comprehensive services*. Washington, DC: Education and Human Services Consortium, Institute for Educational Leadership.

Melton, G. 1983. Children's consent: A Problem in law and social science. In Gary B. Melton, Gerald P. Koocher, and Michael Saks (Eds.), *Children's competence to consent*. New York, NY: Plenum Press.

Mendoza, F., Martorell, R., & Castillo, R. 1989. Health and nutritional status of Mexican-American children. Springfield, VA: National Technical Information Service.

Meredith, C.N., & Frontera, W.R. 1992. Adolescent fitness. In Michael P. Nussbaum and Johanna T. Dwyer (Eds.), *Adolescent medicine: Adolescent nutrition and eating disorders*, 3 (3): 391-404. Philadelphia, PA: Hanley & Belfus, Inc.

Metlife. 1991. The American teacher, 1991--The first year: New teachers' expectations and ideals.

Michigan Catholic Conference Board of Directors. 1987. Teen health and school-based clinics: A statement of the Michigan Catholic Conference board of directors. *Focus* 15, #1.

Millar, H.E. 1975. New approaches to the delivery of health care to adolescents. *Acta Pediatrica Scnadinavica*, 256: 39-45.

Miller, B.C., Card, J.J., Paikoff, R.L. & Peterson, J.L. 1992. *Preventing adolescent pregnancy*. Newbury Park, CA: Sage Publications.

Miller, B.C., Norton, M.C., Jenson, G.O., Lee, T.R., Christopherson, C., & King, P.K. 1993. Pregnancy prevention programs: Impact evaluation of facts & feelings: A home-based video sex education curriculum. *Family Relations*, 42: 392-400.

Miller, K. 1991. School and community-based teen health centers: Michigan's experience. *Clinic News*.

Millstein, S.G. 1988. *The potential of school linked centers to promote adolescent health and development*. Carnegie Council on Adolescent Development: Working Papers Series.

Millstein, S.G., Irwin, C.E., & Brandis, C. 1990. Sociodemographic trends and projections in the adolescent population. In W.R. Hendee (Ed.), *The health of adolescents*, pp. 1-16. San Francisco, CA: Jossey-Bass.

Millstein, S.G., & Litt, I.F. 1990. At the threshold: The developing adolescent. In S. Shirley Feldman and Glen R. Elliott (Eds.), *Adolescent health*, pp. 431-456. Cambridge, MA: Harvard University Press.

Millstein, S.G., Nightingale, E.O., Petersen, A.C., Mortimer, A., & Hamburg, D.A. 1993. Promoting the healthy development of adolescents. *Journal of the American Medical Association*, 269: 1413-1415.

Moll, L. 1991. Why school-based clinics are coming of age. *Pediatric Management*, 24: 19-21.

Monheit, A.C., & Cunningham, P.J., 1992. Children without health insurance. *The Future of Children: U.S. Health Care for Children*, 2(2): 154-170.

Monismith, S.W., Shute, R.E., St. Pierre, R.W. & Alles, W.F., 1984. Opinions of seventh to twelfth graders regarding the effectiveness of pro-and anti-smoking messages. In S. Eioman, J. Wingard, & G. Huba (Eds.), *Drug abuse foundations for a psychosocial approach*, pp. 209-221. New York, NY: Baywood.

Montgomery, K.C., 1990. In Charles Atkin, & Lawrence Wallack (Eds.), *promoting health through entertainment.* Newbury Park, CA: Sage Publications.

Moodie, D.S. 1991. Our children's health: Prospects for the 1990's. *Clinical Pediatrics*, 30: 357-362.

Moody, B., & McKay, L. 1993. PREP: A process, not a recipe. *Educational Leadership*, 51: 28-30.

Moon, M., & Holahan, J. 1992. Can states take the lead in health care reform? *Journal of the American Medical Association*, 268: 1588-1594.

Moore, K.A., Snyder, N.A., & Daly, M. 1992. *Facts at a glance.* Washington, DC: Child Trends.

Moore, K.A., Snyder, N.A., & Halla, C. 1993. *Facts at a glance.* Washington, DC: Child Trends.

Moore, K.A., & Wertheimer, R.F. 1984. Teenage childbearing and welfare. *Family Planning Perspectives*, 16: 285-289.

Moore, N.B., & Davidson, J.K. 1993. *College women and personal goals: Cognitive dimensions that differentiate risk-reduction sexual decisions.* Baltimore, MD: National Center for Family Relations.

Morbidity and Mortality Weekly Report. 1991. Perceptions about sexual behavior: Findings from a national sex knowledge survey - United States, 1989. *Morbidity and Mortality Weekly Report*, 40: 255-259.

Morbidity and Mortality Weekly Report. 1992. Unintentional firearm-related fatalities among children and teenagers - United States, 1982 - 1988. *Morbidity and Mortality Weekly Report*, 41: 442-445.

Morbidity and Mortality Weekly Report. 1994. Health risk behaviors among adolescents who do and do not attend school - United States, 1992. *Morbidity and Mortality Weekly Report*, 43: 129-133.

Morgan, M. 1993. Television and school performance. In Victor C. Strasburger and George A. Comstock (Eds.), *Adolescent medicine: Adolescents and the media*, 4 (3): 607-622. Philadelphia: Hanley & Belfus, Inc.

Morrill, W.A. 1991. *Improving outcomes for children and families at risk: Collaborations which integrate services.* Prepared for the U.S. Department of Education and U.S. Department of Health and Human Services.

Morrill, W.A., & Gerry; M.H. 1990. *Integrating the delivery of services to school-aged children at risk: Toward a description of American experience and experimentation.* Princeton, NJ: Mathtech, Inc.

Morrill, W.A., Reisner, E.R., Chimerine, C.B., & Marks, E.L. 1991. *Collaborations that integrate services for children and families.* Prepared for U.S. Dept. of Education and U.S. Department of Health and Human Services.

Morris, N.M. 1992. Determinants of adolescent initiation of coitus. In Susan M. Coupey and Lorraine V. Klerman (Eds.), *Adolescent medicine: Adolescent sexuality: Preventing unhealthy consequences*, 3 (2): 165-180. Philadelphia, PA: Hanley & Belfus, Inc.

Morrison, D.M., & Shaklee, H. 1990. Poor contraceptive use in the teenage years: Situational and developmental interpretations. In Arlene R. Stiffman and Ronald A. Feldman (Eds.), *Adolescent mental health: Research-practice annual Vol. 4*, pp. 51-69. London: Jessica Kingsley Publishers.

Morse, R.M., & Flavin, D.K. 1992. The definition of alcoholism. *Journal of American Medical Association*, 268: 1012-1014.

Moss, A.J., Allen, K.F., Giovino, G.A., & Mills, S.L. 1992. Recent trends in adolescent smoking, smoking-uptake correlates, and expectations about the future. *Advance Data From the Vital & Health Statistics*, No 221. Hyattsville, MD: National Center for Health Statistics.

Mott, F.L., & Haurin, R.J. 1987. The inter-relatedness of age at first intercourse, early pregnancy, alcohol, & drug use among American adolescents. Unpublished paper: Center for Human Resource Research, The Ohio State University.

Mott, F.L., & Haurin, R.J. 1988. Linkages between sexual activity and alcohol and drug use among American adolescents. *Family Planning Perspectives*, 20: 128-136.

Munger, C.B. 1990. Adolescents and AIDS: Three Michigan physicians reach out to educate youth about AIDS/HIV. *Michigan Medicine*, (February): 16-19.

Murphy, N.T., & Price, D.J. 1988. The influence of self-esteem, parental smoking, and living in a tobacco production region on adolescent smoking behaviors. *Journal of School Health*, 58: 401-405.

Must, A., Jacques, P.F., & Dallal, G.E. 1992. Long-term morbidity and mortality of over weight adolescents: a follow-up of the harvard growth study of 1922 to 1935. *The New England Journal of Medicine*, 32919): 1350-1355.

National Center for Children in Poverty. 1990. *Five million children: A statistical profile of our poorest young citizens.* Columbia University, NY: National Center for Children in Poverty: School of Public Health.

National Center for Clinical Infant Programs. 1992. How community violence affects children, parents, and practitioners. *Public Welfare*, (Fall): 23-35.

National Center for Education in Maternal and Child Health. 1990. *The health of America's youth.* Washington, DC: National Center for Education in Maternal and Child Health.

National Center for Health Statistics. 1984. *Health, United States.* Washington, DC: U.S. Government Printing Office.

National Center on Child Abuse and Neglect. 1988. *Study findings: Study of national incidence and prevalence of child abuse and neglect.* Washington, DC: U.S. Department of Health and Human Services.

National Commission on Children. 1991. *Beyond rhetoric: A new American agenda for children & families.* Washington, DC: U.S. Government Printing Office.

National Commission Against Drunk Driving. 1988. Youth driving without impairment: A community challenge. *Report on the youth impaired driving public hearings.* Washington, DC: National Highway & Traffic Safety Administration.

National Commission for Employment Policy. 1991. *Coordinating federal assistance programs for the economically disadvantaged: Recommendations and background materials.* Special Report #31, October. Washington, DC: National Commission for Employment Policy.

National Conference of Catholic Bishops. 1984. Catholic social teaching and the US economy. *Origins*, 14.

National Conference of Catholic Bishops. 1986. *Economic justice for all.* Washington, DC: United States Catholic Conference, Inc.

National Conference of Catholic Bishops, Administrative Committee. 1988. *Statement to youth on school-based clinics.* Washington, DC: Office of Publishing and Promotion Services, United States Catholic Conference.

National Conference of Catholic Bishops. 1991. Putting children and families first: A Challenge for our Church, nation and world. *Origins*, 21: 393-404.

National Institute on Drug Abuse. 1987. Use of selected drugs among Hispanics, Mexican Americans: *Findings from the Hispanic Health and Nutrition Examination Survey.* Rockville, MD: National Institute on Drug Abuse.

National Institute on Drug Abuse. 1989a. *Highlights of the 1988 National Household Survey onDrug Abuse.* Washington, DC: United States Government Printing Office.

National Institute on Drug Abuse. 1989b. *National Household Survey on drug Abuse: Population Estimates.* Washington, DC: U.S. Government Printing Office.

National Institute on Drug Abuse & U.S. Deptartment of Health and Human Services. 1990. *National household survey on drug abuse main findings,* 1988. Washington, DC: United States Government Printing Office.

National Research Council. 1993. *Understanding child abuse and neglect.* Washington, DC: National Academy Press.

Neff, B.J. 1991. Communication and relationships. In Donald Ratcliff and James A. Davies (Eds.), *Handbook of youth ministry,* pp. 162-177. Birmingham, AL: R.E.P. Books.

Nelson, C. 1991. Office visits by adolescents. *Advance data from vital & health statistics.* Hyattsville, MD: National Center for Health Statistics.

Nelson, D.W. 1991. The Role of Training and Technical Assistance in the Promotion of More Effective Services for Children. In Lisbeth B. Schorr, Deborah Both, and Carol Copple (Eds.), *Effective Services for Young Children: Report of a Workshop,* pp. 80-83. Washington, DC: National Academy Press.

Nelson, J.S. 1985. Faith and adolescents: Insights from psychology and sociology. In John Roberts (Ed.), *Faith maturing: A personal and communal task,* pp. 95-170. Washington, DC: National Federation for Catholic Youth Ministry.

Neuhaus, R. J. 1993. A better choice. *National Review,* August 9, pp. 52-53.

Neumann, C.G. & Jenks, B.H. Obesity. In Melvin D. Levine, William B. Carey, and Allen C. Crocker (Eds.), *Developmental-behavioral pediatrics,* pp. 354-363. Philadelphia, PA: W.B.Saunders Company.

New Futures/Community Connections. 1989. Barrier identification report. *New Futures/Community Connections,* November 15, 1989.

Newacheck, P.W. 1989a. Adolescents with special health needs: Prevalence, severity, and access to health services. *Pediatrics*, 84: 872-881.

Newacheck, P.W. 1989b. Improving access to health services for adolescents from economically disadvantaged families. *Pediatrics*, 84 (6): 1056-1063.

Newacheck, P.W. 1990. Improving access to health care for children, youth, and pregnant women. *Pediatrics*, 86: 626-635.

Newacheck, P.W., & McManus, M.A. 1989. Health insurance status of adolescents in the United States. *Pediatrics*, 84: 699-708.

Newacheck, P.W., McManus, M.A., & Fox, H.B. 1991. Prevalence and impact of chronic illness among adolescents. *Chronic Illness*, 145: 1367-1373.

Newacheck, P.W., Stoddard, J.J., & McManus, M. 1993. Ethnocultural variations in the prevalence and impact of childhood chronic conditions. *Pediatrics*, 91: 10-31-1039.

Newacheck, P.W., & Taylor, W.R. 1992. Childhood chronic illness: Prevalence, severity, and impact. *American Journal of Public Health*, 82: 364-371.

Nicholson, B. 1993. What one school has accomplished: School-based adolescent health care in the 90's. *NAASP Bulletin*, 77: 66-69.

Novack, D., Detering, B., Arnold, R., Forrow, L., Ladinsky, M., & Pezzullo, J.C. 1989. Physicians' attitude toward using deception to resolve difficult ethical problems. *Journal of the American Medical Association*, 261: 2980-2985.

Novello, A. 1988. *Report of the Secretary's Work Group on pediatric HIV infection and diseases*, pp. 17-20. Washington, DC: Department of Health and Human Services.

Novello, A.C, & Shosky, J. 1992. Underage drinking - Laws, loopholes, & enforcement. *Journal of the American Medical Association*, 268: 1391.

Novello, A.C., Shosky, J., & Froehlke, R. 1992. A medical response to violence. *Journal of American Medical Association*, 267: 3007.

Nowinski, J. 1990. *Substance abuse in adolescents and young adults*. New York, NY: W.W. Norton & Company.

Nutter, D.O., Helms, C.M., Whitcomb, M.E., & Weston, W.D. 1991. Restructuring health care in the United States. *Journal of the American Medical Association*, 265: 2516-2520.

O'Carroll, P.W., & Smith, J.C. 1988. Suicide and homicide. In Helen Wallace, George Ryan, and Allan C. Oglesby (Eds.), *Maternal and child health practices*, pp. 583-597. Oakland CA: Third Party Publishing Company.

Oden, S., Kelly, M.A., Ma, Z., & Weikart, D.P. 1992. *Challenging the potential: Programs for talented disadvantaged youth*. Ypsilanti, MI: High/Scope Press.

Offer, D., Ostrov, E., & Howard, K.I. 1991. Disorders of self-image, depression, and suicide. In William R. Hendee (Ed.), *The health of adolescents*, pp. 334-346. San Francisco, CA: Jossey-Bass.

Ohio Bishops. 1986. Ohio Bishops' statement regarding governor's task force on adolescent sexuality and pregnancy. *Focus*, 20, 4: 1-2. Catholic Conference of Ohio.

Olsen, J., Weed, S., Nielsen, A., & Jensen, L. 1992. Student evaluation of sex education programs advocating abstinence. *Adolescence*, 27: 370-380. San Diego, CA: Libra Publishers, Inc.

Olson, T.D., Wallace, C.M., & Miller, B.C. 1984. Primary prevention of adolescent pregnancy: Promoting family involvement through a school curriculum. *Journal of Primary Prevention*, 5: 75-91.

O'Malley, P.M., Johnston, L.D., & Bachman, J.D. 1993. Adolescent substance use and addictions: Epidemiology, current trends, and public policy. In Manuel Schydlower and Peter Rogers (Eds.). *Adolescent medicine: Adolescent substance abuse and addictions*, 4 (2): 227-248. Philadelphia, PA: Hanley & Belfus, Inc.

O'Malley, W.J. 1991. Don't upset the kids. *America*, 165: 190-193.

Ooms, T. 1989. *Integrated approaches to youths' health problems: Federal, state and community roles*. Washington, DC: Family Impact Seminars, The American Association of Marriage and Family Therapy Research and Education Foundation.

Ooms, T., & Hara , S. 1991. *The family-school partnership: A critical component of school reform*. Washington, DC: Family Impact Seminars, The American Association of Marriage and Family Therapy Research and Education Foundation.

Ooms, T., & Hara, S. 1992. *The family-school partnership: A critical component of school reform*. Family Impact Seminars, The American Association of Marriage and Family Therapy Research and Education Foundation.

Ooms, T., Hara, S., & Owen, T. 1992. Service integration and coordination at the family/client level. *Part Three: Is case management the answer?* Washington, DC: Family Impact Seminars, The American Association of Marriage and Family Therapy Research and Education Foundation.

Ooms, T., & Herendeen, L. 1989. *Teenage pregnancy prevention programs: What have we learned?*. Washington, DC: The Family Impact Seminars, The American Association of Marriage and Family Therapy Research and Education Foundation.

Ooms, T., & Owen, T. 1990. *Parents' role in teenage health problems: Allies or adversaries?* Washington, DC: The Family Impact Seminars, The American Association of Marriage and Family Therapy Research and Education Foundation.

Ooms, T., & Owen, T. 1991a. Coordination, collaboration, integration: Strategies for serving families more effectively. *Part One: The federal role.* Washington, DC: Family Impact Seminars, The American Association for Marital and Family Therapy.

Ooms, T., & Owen, T. 1991b. *Promoting adolescent health and well-being through school linked, multi-service, family friendly programs.* Washington, DC: Family Impact Seminars, The American Association of Marriage and Family Therapy Research and Education Foundation.

Ooms, T., & Owen, T. 1991c). *Teenage mothers and the family support act: What works--"carrots" or "sticks"?* Washington, DC: Family Impact Seminars, The American Association of Marriage and Family Therapy Research and Education.

Ooms, T., & Owen, T. 1992. Coordination, collaboration, integration: Strategies for serving families more effectively. *Part Two: State and local initiatives.* Washington, DC: Family Impact Seminar.

Oreskovich, J., & Bensel, R.W. 1991. Maltreatment of adolescents. In William R., Hendee (Ed.), *The health of adolescents*, pp. 347-376. San Francisco, CA: Jossey-Bass Publishing Co.

Orr, M. 1982. Sex education and contraceptive education in United States public high schools. *Family Planning Perspectives*, 14: 304-313.

Ozawa, M.N. 1990. Social policy and out-of-wedlock births to adolescents. In Arlene R. Stiffman and Ronald A. Feldman (Eds.), *Adolescent mental health: Research-practice annual*, pp. 281-299. London: Jessica Kingsley Publishers.

Pacheco, M., Adelsheim, S., Davis, L., Nelson, L. P., Mancha, V., Aime, L., Nelson, P., Derksen, D., & Kaufmann, A. 1991. Innovation, peer teaching, and multidisciplinary collaboration: Outreach from a school-based clinic. *Journal of School Health*, 61: 367-369.

Panzarine, S. (Ed.). 1991. *Promoting the health of adolescents: Proceedings from the 1990 state adolescent health coordinators conference.* Washington, DC: National Center for Education in Maternal and Child Health.

Pascale, A. 1990. School-based clinics. *The Facts*, (June). Washington, DC: Center for Population Options.

Patterson, G.R., DeBaryshe, B.D., & Ramsey, E. 1989. A developmental perspective on antisocial behavior. *American Psychologist*, 44 (2): 329-335.

Paulson, J.A., 1990. Injuries: The leading cause of morbidity and mortality in adolescents. In Victor C. Strasburger, and Donald E. Greydanus (Eds.), *Adolescent medicine: The at-risk adolescent*, 1: 97-112.

Paulson, J. & DiGuiseppi, C. 1995. Adolescent injury prevention in primary care. In Katherine Kaufer Christoffel & Carol W. Runyan (Eds.), *Adolescent medicine: Adolescent injuries: Epidemiology and prevention*, 6 (2): 215-232. Philadelphia, PA: Hanley & Belfus, Inc.

Pentz, M.A., Dwyer, J.H., MacKinnon, D.P., Flay, B.R., Hansen, W.B., Wang, E.Y.I., & Johnson, C.A. 1989. A Multicommunity trial for primary prevention of adolescent drug abuse: Effects on drug use prevalence. *Journal of American Medical Association*, 261: 3259-3266.

Perkin, R.L. 1992. The family in family practice. In Russell J. Sawa (Ed.), *Family Health Care*, pp. 227-238. Newbury Park, CA: Sage Publications.

Perrin, J.M. 1990. Children with special health needs: A United States perspective. *Pediatrics*, 86:1120-1123.

Perry, C.L., Kelder, S.H., Murray, D., & Klepp, K. 1992. Communitywide smoking prevention: Long-term outcomes of the Minnesota Heart Health Program and class of 1989 study. *American Journal of Public Health*, 82: 1210-1216.

Perry, C.L., Telch, M.J., Killen, J., Burke, A., & Maccoby, N. 1983. High school smoking prevention: The relative efficacy of varied treatments and instructors. *Adolescence*, 18: 561-566.

Petersen, A., Compas, B.E., Brooks-Gunn, J.B. Stemmler, M., & Ey, S. 1993. Depression in adolescence. *American Psychologist - Special Issue on Adolescence*, 48: 155-168.

Peterson, J.L., Card, J.J., Eisen, M.B., & Sherman-Williams, B. 1994. Evaluating teenage pregnancy prevention and other social programs: Ten stages of program assessment. *Family Planning Perspectives*, 26: 116-131.

Philliber, S., & Namerow, P.B. 1990. Using the luker model to explain contraceptive use among adolescents. In Arlene R. Stiffman and Ronald A. Feldman (Eds.), *Adolescent mental health research-practice annual Vol. 4*, pp. 71-86. London: Jessica Kingsley Publishers.

Pianta, R.P., Egeland, B.E., & Erickson, M.F. 1989. The antecedents of maltreatment: Results of the mother-child interaction research project. In Dante Cicchetti and Vicki Carlson (Eds.), *Child maltreatment*, pp. 203-253. New York, NY: Cambridge University Press.

Pick de Weiss, S., Atkin, L.C., Gribble, J.N., & Andrade-Palos, P. 1991. Sex, contraception, and pregnancy among adolescents in Mexico City. *Studies in Family Planning*, 22: 74-82.

Pittman, K. & Adams, G. 1988. *Teenage pregnancy: An advocate's guide to the numbers*. Washington, DC: Children's Defense Fund.

Pittman, K.J., Wilson, P.M., Adams-Taylor, S., & Randolph, S. 1992. Making sexuality education and prevention programs relevant for African-American Youth. *Journal of School Health*, 62: 339-344.

Pius XI, Pope. 1931. *Quadragesimo anno*. New York, NY: Barry Vail Corporation.

Place, M.D. 1988. The many faces of AIDS: Some clarifications of the recent debate. *America*, 158: 135-141, 171.

Placier, P. 1992. How "at risk" students plagued a nation: On threat as the warrant for educational policymaking. *Foundations of Education*. Columbia, MO: University of Missouri-Columbia.

Polednak, A.P. 1989. *Racial and ethnic differences in disease*. New York, NY: Oxford University Press.

Polgar, S. 1968. Health. In David L. Sills (Ed.), *International encyclopedia of the social sciences*, Volume 6, pp. 330-336. U.S.A.: Crowell Collier and MacMillan , Inc.

Pollis, C.A. 1985. Value judgments and world views in sexuality education. *Family Relations*, 34: 285-289.

Ponessa, J. 1993. Teaching abstinence: It isn't that simple. *Governing,* (July): 24.

Pontifical Council for the Family, The. 1989. *Marriage and family: Experiencing the Church's teaching in married life.* San Francisco, CA: Ignatius Press.

Posavac, E.J., & Miller, T.Q. 1990. Some problems caused by not having a conceptual foundation for health research: An Illustration from studies of the psychological effects of abortion. *Psychology and Health*, 5: 13-23.

Post, S.G. 1992. Adolescents in a time of AIDS: Preventive education. *America*, 167: 278-282.

Postrado, L.T., & Nicholson, H.J. 1992. Effectiveness in delaying the initiation of sexual intercourse of girls aged 12-14: Two components of the girls incorporated preventing adolescent pregnancy program. *Youth and Society*, 23: 356-379.

Prager, R. 1993. Designing an ethics class. *Educational Leadership*, 51: 32-33.

Press, I. 1982. Witch doctor's legacy: some anthropological implications for the practice of clinical medicine. In Noel J. Curisman and Thomas W. Maretcki (Eds.). *Clinically applied anthropology: Anthropologists in health science settings,* pp. 179-198. Boston, MA: D. Reidel Publishing Co.

Price, J.H., Desmond, S.M., & Smith, D. 1991. A preliminary investigation of inner city adolescents' perceptions of guns. *Journal of School Health*, 61: 255-259.

Price, R., Cioci, M., Penner, W., & Trautlein, B. 1990. *School and community support programs that enhance adolescent health and education.* Washington, DC: Carnegie Council on Adolescent Development.

Prothrow-Stith, D. 1991. *Deadly consequences.* New York, NY: Harper Collins.

Quadrel, M.J., Fischhoff, B., & Davis, W. 1993. Adolescent (in) vulnerability. *American Psychologist - Special Issue on Adolescence*, 48: 102-116.

Quinn, T.C., Glasser, D., & Cannon, R.O. 1988. Human immunodeficiency virus infection among patients attending clinics for sexually transmitted diseases. *New England Journal of Medicine*, 318: 197-203.

Quint, J.C. 1990. Project redirection: Making & measuring a difference. In Arlene R. Stiffman and Ronald A. Feldman (Eds.), *Adolescent mental health: Research practice annual*, pp. 137-157. London: Jessica Kingsley Publishers.

Rabin, J.M., Seltzer, V., & Pollack, S. 1991. The long term benefits of a comprehensive teenage pregnancy program. *Clinical Pediatrics*, 30: 305-309.

Rafferty, Y., & Shinn, M. 1991. The impact of homelessness on children. *American Psychologist*, 46: 1170-1179.

Ramirez, O. 1990. Mexican American children and adolescents. In Jewelle T. Gibbs, Larke Nahme Huang, and associates (Eds.), *Children of color: Psychological inventions with minority youth*. San Francisco, CA: Jossey Bass.

Ratcliff, D., & Davies, J.A. (Eds.). 1991. *Handbook of youth ministry*. Birmingham, AL: R.E.P. Books.

Rauenhorst, J.M. 1972. Followup of young women who attempt suicide. *Diseases of the Nervous System*, 33: 792-797.

Raunikar, R.A., & Strong, W.B. 1991. The status of adolescent fitness. In Paul G. Dyment (Ed.), *Adolescent medicine: Sports and the adolescent*, 2 (1): 65-78. Philadelphia, PA: Hanley & Belfus, Inc.

Ravoira, L., & Cherry, A.L. 1992. *Social bonds & teen pregnancy*. Westport, CN: Praeger.

Reardon, D.C. 1990. *Aborted women: Silent no more*. Westchester, IL: Crossway Books.

Rees, J.M., & Office of Maternal and Child Health. 1988. Nutritional issues in adolescent health. *Information bulletin: Youth 2000*. Rockville, MD: United States Department of Health and Human Services.

Reiss, M. 1994. The subject of sex. *The Tablet*. February 19: 210-211.

Resnick, M.D., Chambliss, S.A., & Blum, R.W. 1993. Health and risk behaviors of urban adolescent males involved in pregnancy. *The Journal of Contemporary Human Services*, (June): 366-374.

Rich, V. 1993. Poland: Abortion. *The Lancet*, 34: 1083-1084.

Richardson, R.A. 1991. Bittersweet connections: Informal social networks as sources of support and interference for adolescent mothers. *Family Relations*, 40: 430-434.

Rickert, V.I., Gottlieb, A., & Jay, M.S. 1990. A comparison of three clinic-based AIDS education programs on female adolescents' knowledge, attitudes, and behavior. *Journal of Adolescent Health Care*, 11: 298-303.

Rickert, V.I., Jay, M.S., & Gottlieb, A. 1991. Effects of a Peer-counseled AIDS education program on knowledge, attitudes, and satisfaction of adolescents. *Journal of Adolescent Health*, 12: 38-43.

Riessman, J. 1991. School-based and school-linked clinics. Newsletter from Center for Population Options. Washington, DC: The Center for Population Options.

Riley, W.A., & Schneckenburger, W.A. 1991. The Maryland experience and a practical proposal to expand existing models in ambulatory primary care. *Journal of The American Medical Association*, 266: 1118-1122.

Rimsza, M.E., & Niggemann, E.H. 1982. Medical evaluation of sexually abused children: A review of 311 cases. *Pediatrics*, 69: 8-14.

Risser, W.L. 1991. Epidemiology of sports injuries in adolescents. In Paul G. Dyment (Ed.), *Adolescent medicine: Sports and the adolescent*, 2 (1): 109-124. Philadelphia, PA: Hanley & Belfus, Inc.

Rivara, F.P. 1985. Fatal and nonfatal injuries to children and adolescents in the United States. *Pediatrics*, 76: 567-573.

Roach, J.R. 1988. Statement of school-based clinics - unpublished paper. St. Paul, MN: Archdiocese of St. Paul and Minneapolis.

Robenstine, C. 1993. Combating a killer, HIV education at the secondary level: An urgent necessity. *NASSP Bulletin*, 77: 9-16.

Roberts, R.N., Wasik, B., Casto, G., & Ramey, C.T. 1991. Family support in the home: Programs, policy, and social change. *American Psychologist*, 46: 131-137.

Rockefeller, J.D., IV. 1991. A call for action: The Pepper Commission's blueprint for health care reform. *Journal of the American Medical Association*, 265: 2507-2510.

Rodman, H. 1990. Legal and social dilemmas of adolescent sexuality. In John Bancroft and June Cachover Reinisch (Eds.), *Adolescence and puberty*, pp. 254-268. New York, NY: Oxford University Press.

Rodman, H., Lewis, S.H., & Griffith, S.B. 1984. *The sexual rights of adolescents: Competence, vulnerability, and parental control.* New York, NY: Columbia University Press.

Rogers, E.M., & Storey, J.D. 1987. Communication campaigns. *Handbook of communication science*, pp. 817-846. Beverly Hills, CA: Sage Publications.

Rogers, J.A., & Elliott, B.A. 1989. The physician's role in adolescent health education. *Minnesota Medicine*, 72: 461-463, 466.

Rogers, P.D., & Adger, H. 1993. Alcohol and adolescents. In Manuel Schydlower and Peter Rogers (Eds.), *Adolescent medicine: Adolescent substance abuse and addictions*, 4 (2): 295-304. Philadelphia, PA: Hanley & Belfus, Inc.

Roosa, M.W., & Christopher, F.S. 1990. Evaluation of an abstinence-only adolescent pregnancy prevention program: A replication. *Family Relations*, 39: 363-367.

Roosa, M.W., & Christopher, F.S. 1992. A response to Thiel and McBride: Scientific criticism or obscuratism? *Family Relations*, 41: 468-469.

Roosmalen, E.H., & McDaniel, S.A. 1992. Adolescent smoking intentions: Gender differences in peer context. *Adolescence*, 27: 87-105.

Ropp, L., Visintainer, P., Uman, J., & Treloar, D. 1992. Death in the city: An American childhood tragedy. *Journal of the American Medical Association*, 267: 59-64.

Rosen, D.S. 1994. Transition from pediatric to adult-oriented health care for the adolescent with chronic illness or disability. In Robert T. Brown and Susan M. Coupey (Eds.), *Adolescent medicine: Chronic and disabling disorders*, 5 (2): 241-248. Philadelphia, PA: Hanley & Belfus, Inc.

Rosen, D.S., Xiangdong, M., & Blum, R. 1990. Adolescent health: Current trends and critical issues. In Victor C. Strasburger and Donald E. Greydanus (Eds.), *Adolescent medicine: The at-risk adolescents*, 1 (1): 15-31. Philadelphia, PA: Hanley & Belfus, Inc.

Rosenbaum, S., Huges, D., Harris, P., & Liu, J. 1992. *Special report: Children and health insurance.* Washington, DC: Health Division, Children's Defense Fund.

Rosenbaum, S., Layton, C., & Liu , J. 1991. *The health of America's children.* Washington,DC: The Children's Defense Fund.

Rosenberg, M.L., Mercy, J.A., & Houk, V.N. 1991. Guns and adolescent suicide. *Journal of the American Medical Association*, 266: 3030.

Rosenberg, M.L., Rodriguez, J.G., & Chorba, T.L. 1990. Childhood injuries: Where we are. Pediatrics, 86: 1084-1091.

Ross, J.G., & Gilbert, G. 1985. The National Youth and Fitness Study: A summary of findings. *Journal of Physical Education, Recreation, and Dance*, 56: 45-50.

Ross, J.G., & Pate, R. 1987. A summary of findings of the National Children and Youth Fitness Study II. *Journal of Physical Education, Recreation, and Dance*, 60: 51-56.

Rowlatt, G.W., Jr. 1989. *Pastoral care with adolescents in crisis*. Louisville, KY: Westminster/John Knox Press.

Roybal, E. 1991. The 'US Health Act': Comprehensive reform for a caring America. *Journal of the American Medical Association*, 265: 2545-2548.

Rubin, R.L. 1986. Assisting adolescents toward mental health. *Nursing Clinics of North America*, 21: 439-450.

Runyan, C.W., & Gerken, E.A. 1989. Epidemiology and Prevention of adolescent injury: A review and research agenda. *Journal of the American Medical Association*, 262: 2273-2279.

Runyan, C.W., & Gerken, E.A. 1991. Injuries. In William R. Hendee (Ed.), *The health of adolescents*, pp. 302-333. San Francisco, CA: Jossey Bass.

Russo, N.F. 1992. Psychological aspects of unwanted pregnancy and its resolution. In J. Douglas Butler and David F. Walbert, (Eds.), *Abortion, medicine, and the law*, pp. 593-628. New York, NY: Facts on File.

Ryan, K. 1993. Mining the values in the curriculum. *Educational Leadership*, 51: 16-18.

Ryan, S.A. & Irwin, C.E. 1992. Risk behaviors. In Stanford B. Friedman, Martin Fisher, and S. Kenneth Schonberg (Eds.), *Comprehensive adolescent health care*, pp. 787-794. St. Louis, MO: Quality Medical Publishing, Inc.

Sahler, O.J.Z., & McAnarney, E.R. 1981. *The child from three to eighteen*. St. Louis, MO: Mosby-Year Book.

Sanders, J.M. 1988a. Case profile: The hidden agenda. *Adolescent Wellness*, 1:3.

Sanders, J.M. 1988b. Case profile: Treating the symptoms. *Adolescent Wellness,* 1:3.

Sanders, J.M. 1989. Case profile: An atypical adolescent suicide. *Adolescent Wellness,* 1:9.

Santelli, J., Alexander, M., Farmer, M., Papa, P., Johnson, T., Rosenthal, B., & Hotra, D. 1992. Bringing parents into school clinics: Parent attitudes toward school clinics and contraception. *Journal of Adolescent Health,* 13: 269-274.

Sarason, S.B., Carroll, C.F., Maton, K., Cohen, S., & Lorentz, E. 1977. *Human services and resource networks: Rationale, possibilities, and public policy.* Washington, DC: Jossey-Bass.

Sargent, J. 1992. Family variations. In Melvin D. Levine, William B. Carey, and Allen C. Crocker (Eds.), *Developmental-behavioral pediatrics,* pp.109-116. Philadelphia, PA: W.B.Saunders Company.

Saterlie, M.E. 1988. A community-based values program. *Educational Leadership,* 54: 34-37.

Sawa, R.J. 1992a. Expanding our horizons: Visions of the future. In Russell J. Sawa (Ed.), *Family health care,* pp. 239-257. Newbury Park, CA: Sage Publications.

SAWA, R.J. 1992B. Paradigm shift: toward A New vision of family medicine. In Russell J. Sawa (Ed.), *Family health care,* pp. 1-5. Newbury Park, CA: Sage Publications.

Saxe, L.M., Cross, T., & Silverman, N. 1986. Children's mental health: Problems and services. *Report by the Office of Technology Assessment.* Durham, NC: Duke University Press.

Scales, P. 1982. Values' role in sexuality education. *Planned Parenthood Review,* 2: 6-8.

Scales, P. 1983. Sense and nonsense about sexuality education: A rejoinder to the shornacks' critical view. *Family Relations,* 32: 287-295.

Schaefer, R.T., & Lamm, R.P. 1992. *Sociology.* New York, NY: McGraw-Hill, Inc.

Schamess, S. 1993. The search for love: Unmarried adolescent mothers' views of, and relationships with, men. *Adolescence,* 28: 425-437.

Schindler-Rainman, E.R. 1981. Toward collaboration--Risks we need to take. *Journal of Voluntary Research Action*, 10: 120-127.

Schinke, S.P., Botvin, G., & Orlandi, M.A. 1991. *Substance abuse in children and adolescents: Evaluation and intervention.* Newbury Park, CA: Sage Publications.

Schlesinger, M.J., & Eisenberg, L. (Eds.). 1990. *Children in a changing health system: Assessments and proposals for reform.* Baltimore, MD: The Johns Hopkins University Press.

Schoonmaker, R. 1983. A teenage view of cigarette smoking. *Connecticut Medicine*, 47: 705-707.

Schopler, J.H. 1987. Interorganizational groups: Origins, structure, and outcomes. *Academy of Management Review*, 12: 702-713.

Schorr, L.B., & Both, D. 1991. Attributes of effective services for young children: A brief survey of current knowledge and its implications for program and policy development. In Lisbeth B. Schorr, Deborah Both, and Carol Copple (Eds.), *Effective services for young children: Report of a workshop*, pp. 23-47. Washington, DC: National Academy Press.

Schorr, L.B., Both, D., & Copple, C. (Eds.) 1991. *Effective services for young children: Report of a workshop.* Washington, DC: National Academy Press.

Schorr, L.B., & Schorr, D. 1988. *Within our reach: Breaking the cycle of disadvantage.* New York, NY: Doubleday.

Schubert, R.F., & Gates, M. 1990. *Report on the nationwide project--Making the grade: A report card on American youth.* Washington, DC: National Collaboration for Youth.

Schydlower, M., & Shafer, M.A. 1990. Chlamydia trachomatis infections in adolescents. In Manuel Schydlower and Mary-Ann Shafer (Eds.). *Adolescent medicine: AIDS and other sexually transmitted diseases*, 1 (3): 615-628. Philadelphia, PA: Hanley & Belfus, Inc.

Select Committee on Children, Youth, and Families. 1992. *A decade of denial: teens and AIDS in America (Summary).* United States House of Representatives.

Select Panel for the Promotion of Child Health. 1981a. *Better health for children: A national survey.* Washington, DC: United States Government Printing Office.

Select Panel for the Promotion of Child Health. 1981b. *Better health for children: A national survey*, Volume 3. Washington DC: United States Government Printing Office.

Services Integration for Families and Children in Crisis. 1991. *Services integration for families and children in crisis*. Washington, DC: Department of Health and Human Services Office of Inspector General.

Services Integration Pilot Projects. 1989. *An evaluative report from Arizona, Florida, Maine, Oklahoma, South Carolina*. Columbia, SC: State Reorganization Commission.

Services Integration: A Twenty Year Retrospective. 1991. *Services integration: A twenty-year retrospective*. Washington, DC: Office of Inspector General Health and Human Services.

Setterberg, S.R. 1992. Suicidal behavior and suicide. In Stanford B. Friedman, Martin Fisher, and S. Kenneth Schonberg (Eds.), *Comprehensive adolescent health care*, pp. 862-902. St. Louis, MO: Quality Medical Publishing, Inc.

Shaffer, D. 1988. Alcohol/substance abuse and depression. *Adolescent Wellness Newsletter*, 1. Lyndhurst, NJ: Health Learning Systems Inc.

Shaffer, D. 1989. Prevention of adolescent suicide and post suicide intervention. *Adolescent Wellness Newsletter*, 1. Lyndhurst, NJ: Health Learning Services Inc.

Shagle, S.C., & Barber, B.K. 1993. Effects of family, marital, and parent-child conflict on adolescent self-derogation and suicidal ideation. *Journal of Marriage and the Family*, 55: 964-974.

Sheeran, P.J. 1993. *Ethics in public administration: A philosophical approach.* New York, NY: Praeger.

Sheeran, P.J. 1987. *Women, society, the state, and abortion: A structuralist analysis*. New York, NY: Praeger.

Sheils, J. F., & Wolfe, P.R. 1992. The role of private health insurance in children's health care. *The Future of Children: U.S. Health Care for Children*, 2: 115-133.

Sheley, J.F., McGee, Z.T., & Wright, J.D. 1992. Gun-related violence in and around inner-city schools. *American Journal of the Diseases of Children*, 146: 289-294.

Shelton, C.M. 1989. *Morality and the adolescent: A pastoral psychology approach.* New York, NY: Crossroad.

Shiffrin, S.H. 1993. Alcohol and cigarette advertising: A legal primer. In Victor C. Strasburger and George A. Comstock (Eds.), *Adolescent medicine: Adolescents and the media*, 4 (3): 623-634. Philadelphia: Hanley & Belfus, Inc.

Shine, W. 1992. Affluence. In Stanford B. Friedman, Martin Fisher, and S. Kenneth Schonberg (Eds.), *Comprehensive adolescent health care*, pp. 688-691. St. Louis, MO: Quality Medical Publishing, Inc.

Shisslak, C.M., Craso, M., & Neal, M.E. 1990. Prevention of eating disorders among adolescents. *American Journal of Health Promotion*, 5: 100-106.

Shornack, L.L., & Shornack, E.M. 1982a. Reply to Kirkendall. *Family Relations*, 31: 546.

Shornack, L.L., & Shornack, E.M. 1982b. The new sex education and the sexual revolution: A critical view. *Family Relations*, 31: 532-544.

Shorter, E. 1992. Recent changes in family life and new challenges in primary care. In Russell J. Sawa (Ed.), *Family Health Care*, pp. 9-17. Newbury Park, CA: Sage Publications.

Signorielli, N. 1993. *Mass media images and impact on health: A sourcebook.* Westport, CT: Greenwood Press.

Sikand, A., & Fisher, M. 1992. The role of barrier contraceptives in prevention of pregnancy and disease in adolescents. *Adolescent medicine: Adolescent sexuality: Preventing unhealthy consequences*, 3 (2): 223-240.

Silber, T.J., & Rosenthal, J.L. 1986. Usefulness of a review of systems questionnaire in the assessment of the hospitalized adolescent. *Journal of Adolescent Health Care*, 7: 49-52.

Simmons, P.D. 1992. Religious approaches to abortion. In J. Douglas Butler and David F. Walbert (Eds.), *Abortion, medicine, and the law*, pp. 712-730. New York, NY: Facts On File.

Simons, J.M., Finlay, B., & Yang, A. 1991. *The adolescent and young adult fact book.* Washington, DC: Children's Defense Fund.

Sjoberg, G., Williams, N., Gill, N., & Himmel, K.F. 1995. Family Life and Racial and Ethnic Diversity: An Assessment of Communitarianism, Liberalism, and Conservatism. *Journal of Family Issues*, 16 (3): 246-274.

Skaff, L.F. 1988. Child maltreatment coordinating committees for effective service delivery. Child Welfare, 67: 217-230.

Skjeldestad, F.E., & Borgan, J. 1994. Trends in induced abortion during the 12 years since legalization in Norway. *Family Planning Perspective*, 26: 73-76.

Slade, J. 1993. Adolescent nicotine use and dependence. In Manuel Schydlower and Peter Rogers (Eds.), *Adolescent medicine: Adolescent substance abuse and addictions*, 4 (2): 295-304. Philadelphia, PA: Hanley & Belfus, Inc.

Slinski, M. D. 1990. Building communities of support for families in poverty. Massachusetts University, Amherst: Cooperative Extension Service. Paper presented at the Eastern Symposium on Building Family Strengths, University Park, PA on April 17-20, 1990.

Sloan, J.H., Kellermann, A.L., Reay, D.T., Ferris, J.A., Koepsell, T., Rivara, F.P., Rice, C., Gray, L., & LoGerfo, J. 1988. Handgun regulations, crime, assaults, and homicide: A tale of two cities. *The New England Journal of Medicine*, 319: 1256-1262.

Small, S.A., & Kerns, D. 1993. Unwanted sexual activity among peers during early and middle adolescence: Incidence and risk factors. *Journal of Marriage and the Family*, 55: 941-952.

Smith, G.S. & Brenner, R.A. 1995. The changing risks of drowning for adolescents in the U.S. and effective control strategies. In Katherine Kaufer Christoffel & Carol W. Runyan (Eds.), *Adolescent medicine: Adolescent injuries: Epidemiology and prevention*, 6 (2): 153-170. Philadelphia, PA: Hanley & Belfus, Inc.

Snyder, L. 1989. Health care needs of the adolescent. *Annals of Internal Medicine*, 110: 930-935.

Snyder, W. 1992. Seeing the troubled adolescent in context: Family systems theory and practice. In Wendy Snyder and Thedora Ooms (Eds.), *Empowering families, helping adolescents: Family-centered treatment of adolescents with alcohol drug abuse, and mental health problems*, pp. 13-37. Rockville, MD: United States Department of Health and Human Services.

Snyder, W., & Ooms, T. 1992. Introduction and overview. In Wendy Snyder and Theodora Ooms (Eds). *Empowering families, helping adolescents: Family centered treatment of adolescents with alcohol, drug abuse, and mental health problems*, pp. 1-10. Rockville, MD: United States Department of Health and Human Services.

Speckhard, A. 1987. *The psycho-social aspects of stress following abortion.* Kansas City, MO: Sheed & Ward.

Speckhard, A.C. & Rue, V.M. 1992. Postabortion syndrome: An emerging public health concern. *Journal of Social Issues*, 48:95-119.

Spivak, H. 1991. Dying is no accident: Adolescents, violence and intentional injury. In Susan Panzarine (Ed.), *Promoting the health of adolescents: Proceedings from the 1990 State Adolescent Health Coordinators Conference*, pp. 53-58. Washington, DC: National Center for Education in Maternal and Child Health.

Spohn, W.C. 1988. AIDS and the United States Catholic Church. *America*, 158: 142-146.

Stack, S. 1994. The effect of geographic mobility on premarital sex. *Journal of Marriage and the Family*, 56 (1): 204-205.

Stanton, W.R., & Silva, P.A. 1991. School achievement as an independent prediction of smoking in childhood & early adolescence. *Health Education Journal*, 50: 84-88.

Staton, J., Ooms, T., & Owens, T. 1991. Family resource, support, and parent education programs: The power of a preventive approach. *Family Impact Seminars*, October 25, 1991.

Steinberg, L. 1990. Autonomy, conflict and harmony in the family relationship. In S. S. Feldman and G. R. Elliot (Eds.), *At the threshold: The developing adolescent*, pp. 255-276. Cambridge, MA: Harvard University Press.

Steinglass, P. 1992. Family systems theory and medical illness. In Russell J. Sawa (Ed.), *Family health care*, pp. 18-29. Newbury Park, CA: Sage Publications.

Steinhauer, P.D. 1991. *The least detrimental alternative: A systematic guide to case planning and decision making for children in care.* Toronto, Ontario: University of Toronto Press.

Stevens-Simon, C., & Reichert, S. 1994. Sexual abuse, adolescent pregnancy, and child abuse: A developmental approach to an intergenerational cycle. *Archives of Pediatrics and Adolescent Medicine*, 148: 23-28.

Stier-Adler, E., & Merdinger, J.M. 1990. Schools and systems: Policies and programs for pregnant & parenting adolescents. In Arlene R. Stiffman and Ronald A. Feldman (Eds.), *Adolescent mental health: A research-practice annual*, pp. 173-188. London: Jessica Kingsley Publishers.

Stiffman, A.R., & Feldman, R.A. (Eds.). 1990. *Advances in adolescent mental health: A research-practice annual Vol. 4.* London: Jessica Kingsley Publishers.

Strasburger, V.C. 1986a. Does television affect learning and school performance? *Pediatrician*, 13: 141-147.

Strasburger, V.C. 1986b. Prevention of adolescent drug abuse: Why "just say no" just won't work. *Journal of Pediatrics*, 114 (4): 676-681.

Strasburger, V.C. 1989. The adolescent in contemporary western society. In Adele D. Hofman and Donald E. Greydanus (Eds.), *Adolescent medicine*, pp. 3-7. Norwalk, CT: Appleton and Lange.

Strasburger, V.C. 1990. Television and adolescents: Sex, drugs, rock 'n' roll. In Victor C. Strasburger and Donald E. Greydanus (Eds.), *Adolescent medicine: The at-risk adolescent,* 1 (1): 161-194. Philadelphia, PA: Hanley & Belfus, Inc.

Strasburger, V.C. 1992. Electronic media. In Melvin D. Levine, William B. Carey, and Allen C. Crocker (Eds.), *Developmental-behavioral pediatrics*, pp. 171-177. Philadelphia, PA: W.B.Saunders Company.

Strasburger, V.C. 1993. Children, adolescents, and the media: Five crucial issues. In Victor C. Strasburger and George A. Comstock (Eds.), *Adolescent medicine: Adolescents and the media*, 4 (3): 479-494. Philadelphia: Hanley & Belfus, Inc.

Straus, M. 1992. Social stress and marital violence in a national sample of American families. In Murray A. Straus and Richard J. Gelles (Eds.), *Physical violence in American families: risk factors and adaptations to violence in 8,145 families*, pp. 181-201. New Brunswick, NJ: Transaction Publishers.

Straus, M.A., & Gelles, R.J. 1992. How violent are American families? Estimates from National Family Violence resurvey and other studies. In Murray A. Straus and Richard J. Gelles (Eds.), *Physical violence in American families: Risk factors and adaptations to violence in 8,145 families*, pp. 95-112. New Brunswick, NJ: Transaction Publishers.

Straus, M.A., & Smith, C. 1992. Family patterns and child abuse. In Murray A. Straus and Christine Smith (Eds.), *Physical violence in American families: Risk factors and adaptations to violence in 8,145 families*, pp. 245-262. New Brunswick, NJ: Transaction Publishers.

Stravinskas, P.M.J. 1993. *Catholic dictionary.* Huntington, IN: Our Sunday Visitor, Inc.

Strong, W.B. 1994. Preparticipation physical examination: It should be required, Editorial. *Archives of Pediatrics and Adolescent Medicine*, 148: 99-100.

Stroul, B.A., & Friedman, R.M. 1986. *A system of care for severely emotionally disturbed children and youth.* Washington, DC: CASSP Technical Assistance Center.

Stroul, B.A., & Friedman, R.M. 1988a. Principles for a system of care: Special report on caring for severely emotionally disturbed children. *Children Today*, 17: 11-15.

Stroul, B.A., & Friedman, R.M. 1988b. Putting principles into practice. *Children Today*, July-August: 15-17.

Stuart, I.R., & Wells, C.F. 1982. Pregnancy in adolescence. New York, NY: Van Nostrand Reinhold.

Supplement. 1990. Child health in 1990: The United States compared to Canada, England and Wales, France, the Netherlands, and Norway. Proceedings of a Conference, Washington, DC, March 18-19, 1990. *Pediatrics*, 86.

Support Center for School Based Clinics. 1991. *Clinic News*, 7.

Swandener, E.B. 1990. Children and families 'at risk': Etiology, critique, and alternative paradigms. *Educational Foundations*, 4: 17-39.

Symons, C.W., & Gascoigne, J.L. 1990. The Nation's health objectives - A means to school-wide fitness advocacy. *Journal of Physical Education, Recreation, and Dance*, 61(August): 59-63.

Szasz, T. 1961. *The myth of mental illness.* New York, NY: Hoeber-Harper.

Takanish, R. 1993. The opportunities of adolescence - Research, Interventions, and policy: introduction to the special issue. *American Psychologist - Special issue on Adolescence*, 48: 85-87.

Target 2000. 1990. Healthier youth by the year 2000. *Newsletter of the American Medical Association's Project Target 2000*, 1: 1-8.

Thiel, K.S., & McBride, D. 1992. Comments on an evaluation of an abstinence - Only adolescent pregnancy prevention program. *Family Relations*, 41: 465-467.

Thieman, A.A., & Dale, P.W. 1992. Family preservation services: Problems of measurement and assessment of risk. *Family Relations*, 41: 186-191.

Thompson, L.S. (Ed.) 1991. *The forgotten child in health care: Children in the juvenile justice system.* Washington, DC: National Center for Education in Maternal and Child Health.

Tishler, C.L. 1992. Adolescent suicide: Assessment of Risk, prevention and treatment. In Robert T. Brown and Barbara A. Cromer (Eds.), *Adolescent medicine: Psychosocial issues in adolescents*, 3 (1): 51-59. Philadelphia, PA: Hanley & Belfus, Inc.

Todd, J., Seekins, S.V., Krichbaum, J.A., & Harvey, L.K. 1991. Health access America--Strengthening the U.S. health care system. *Journal of the American Medical Association*, 265: 2503.

Tolan, P. & Guerra, N. 1994. *What works in reducing adolescent violence: An empirical review of the field.* Boulder, CO: The Center for the Study and Prevention of Violence.

Tolmas, H.C. 1986. A patient survey helped me get through to teenagers. *Contemporary Pediatrics*, 47-50: 52.

Trafford, A. 1992. Violence as a public health crisis: Health care professionals are out to change behavior that leads to "gun abuse." *Public Welfare,* Fall: 16-17.

Turner, L. 1993. Eight cities fighting teen drinking with dose of creativity. *Nation's Cities Weekly*, pp. 4-5.

Turner, V. 1969. *The ritual process: Structure and anti-structure.* Ithaca, NY: Cornell University.

Tyack, D. 1992. Health and social services in public schools: Historical perspectives. *The Future of Children*, Spring: 20-31.

United States Catholic Bishops. 1981. Health and health care. *Pastoral Letter.* Washington, DC: United States Catholic Conference, Inc.

United States Catholic Bishops. 1987. United States Bishops statement on school-based clinics. *Origins,* 17: 433-441.

United States Catholic Conference. 1983. The holy see to all persons, institutions and authorities concerned with the mission of the family in today's world. *Charter of the Rights of the Family, October 22, 1983.* Washington, DC: United States Catholic Conference.

United States Catholic Conference. 1990. *A century of social teaching: A common heritage, a continuing challenge.* Washington, DC: United States Catholic Conference.

United States Catholic Conference. 1991. *Putting children and families first: A challenge for our church, nation, and world.* Washington, DC: United States Catholic Conference Office of Publishing and Promotional Services.

United States Catholic Conference. 1993. *A framework for comprehensive health care reform: Protecting human life, promoting human dignity, pursuing the common good.* Washington, DC: United States Catholic Conference.

United States Congress, Office of Technology Assessment. 1990. *Indian adolescent mental health.* Washington, DC: United States Government Printing Office.

United States Congress, Office of Technology Assessment. 1991a. *Adolescent health - Volume I: Summary and policy options.* Washington, DC: United States Government Printing Office.

United States Congress, Office of Technology Assessment. 1991b. *Adolescent health - Volume II: Background and the effectiveness of selected prevention and treatment services.* Washington, DC: United States Government Printing Office.

United States Congress, Office of Technology Assessment. 1991c. *Adolescent health - Volume III: Crosscutting issues in the delivery of health and related services.* Washington, DC: United States Government Printing Office.

United States Department Health and Human Services and Centers for Disease Control. 1990. Advance report of final natality statistics. *Monthly Vital Statistics Report* 39. Washington, DC: United States Government Printing Office.

United States Department of Health & Human Services, Centers for Disease Control, & National Center for Health Statistics. 1990. *Vital and health statistics: Health of black and white Americans 1985-1987.* Hyattsville, MD: United States Government Printing Office.

United States Department of Transportation and National Highway Traffic Administration, & National Center for Statistics and Analysis. 1989. *Drunk driving facts.* Washington, DC: United States Government Printing Office.

United States Public Health Service. 1993. *Progress report for: Adolescents and young adults.* Washington, DC: United States Public Health Services.

United States Public Health Service. 1994. *Reducing teenage pregnancy increases life options for youth.* Washington, DC: United States Public Health Service.

Upton, J.A. 1991. Father, I'm pregnant: What do you suggest? *Commonweal,* 118: 217-219.

Vanderschmidt, H.F., Lang, J.M., Knight-Williams, V., & Vanderschmidt, G.F. 1993. Risks among inner-city young teens: The prevalence of sexual activity, violence, drugs, and smoking. *Journal of Adolescent Health,* 14: 282-288.

Vatican, The 1983. *Charter of the rights of the family.* Washington, DC: United States Catholic Conference Office of Publishing and Promotion Service.

Vatican Council II. 1965. *Gaudium et spes: Pastoral constitution on the Church in the modern world.* Boston, MA: St. Paul Editions.

Vaughan, H.P. 1990. *Canonical variatiates of post abortion syndrome.* Portsmouth, NH: Institute for Pregnancy Loss.

Vaughan, V.C., & Litt, I. 1990a. Early adolescence. *Child and Adolescent development: Clinical implications.* Philadelphia, PA: W.B. Saunder Company.

Vaughan, V.C., & Litt, I. 1990b. Middle adolescence. *Child and adolescent development: Clinical implications.* Philadelphia, PA: W.B. Saunder Company.

Vaughan, V.C., & Litt, I. 1990c). Late adolescence. *Child and adolescent development: Clinical implications.* Philadelphia, PA: W.B. Saunder Company.

Vaughan, V.C., & Litt, I.F. 1990d). *Child & adolescent development: Clinical implications.* Philadelphia, PA: W.B. Saunder Company.

Verbrugge, H.P. 1990a. Child health in 1990: The United States compared to Canada, England and Wales, France, the Netherlands, and Norway. Proceedings of a Conference, Washington, DC., March 18 and 19, 1990. *Pediatrics*, 86: 6.

Verbrugge, H.P. 1990b. Children with special needs in the Netherlands: Impaired hearing, adolescent, pregnancy, and myelomeningocele. *Pediatrics*, 86: 1117-1120.

Vernon, M.E.L., & Seymore, C. 1987. Communicating with adolescents in alternative health care sites. *Seminars in Adolescent Medicine*, 3: 115-120.

Vernon, M.E.L., & Seymore, C. 1990. Antecedents and 'predictors' of adolescent pregnancy. In Arlene R. Stiffman and Ronald A. Feldman (Eds.), *Adolescent mental health: Research-practice annual Vol. 4*, pp. 109-119. London: Jessica Kingsley Publishers.

Vincent, M.L., Clearie, A.F., & Schluchter, M.D. 1987. Reducing adolescent pregnancy through school and community-based education. *Journal of American Medical Association*, 257: 3382-3386.

Violato, C. 1992. History of adolescence. In Stanford B. Friedman, Martin Fisher, and S. Kenneth Schonberg (Eds.), *Comprehensive adolescent health care*, 3-6. St. Louis, MO: Quality Medical Publishing, Inc.

Vital Statistics of the United States 1985. 1987. *Mortality*. Washington, DC: United States Government Printing Office.

Voydanoff, P. 1992. Human services integration: A background paper. Unpublished paper, University of Dayton.

Voydanoff, P., & Donnelly, B.W. 1990. *Adolescent sexuality and pregnancy*. Newbury Park, CA: Sage Publications.

Wagner, K.D., & Wagner, R.F. 1985. Impact of acne on sexuality. *Medical aspects of human sexuality*, 19: 252-255.

Walker, J.A., Harris, L., Blum, R., Schneider, & Resnick, 1990. *Outlooks and insights: Understanding rural adolescents*. St. Paul, MN: University of Minnesota.

Wallace, H.M., Ryan, G., & Oglesby, A.C. (Eds.). 1988. *Maternal and child health practices*. Oakland, CA: Third Party Publishing Company.

Wallack, L. 1990. Mass media and health promotion: Promise, problem, and challenge. In Charles Atkin, and Lawrence Wallack (Eds.), *Mass communication and public health complexities and conflicts.* Newbury Park, CA: Sage Publications.

Wallack, L., Grube, J.W., Madden, P.A., & Breed, W. 1990. Portrayals of alcohol on prime-time television. *Journal Studies on Alcohol*, 51: 428-437.

Wang, M.C. & Gordon, E.W. (Eds.). 1994. *Educational Resilience in Inner-City America: Challenges and Prospects.* Hillsdale, NJ: Lawrence Erlbaum Associates, Publishers.

Warren, C., & Neer, M. 1986. Family sex communication orientation. *Journal of Applied Communication Research*, 14: 86-107.

Waszak, C., & Neidell, S. 1991. *School-based and school-linked clinics.* Washington, DC: The Center for Population Options.

Watkins, T., & Rall, S. 1986. *Information on school based health clinics.* Lansing, MI: Catholic Charities, Diocese of Lansing.

Watzman, N. 1990. When sex ed becomes chastity class. *Utne Reader*, 40: 92-97.

Wauchope, B., & Straus, M. 1990. Physical punishment and physical abuse of American children: Incidence rates by age, gender, and occupational class. In M.A. Straus and R.J. Gelles (Eds.), *Physical violence in American families: Risk Factors and adaptations to violence in 8,145 families*, pp. 133-150. New Brunswick, NJ: Transaction Books.

Weiner, M.E. 1990. *Human services management: Analysis and applications, Second edition.* Belmont, CA: Wadsworth Publishing Co.

Weisfeld, V.D. (Ed.). 1989. A summary of Robert Wood Johnson Foundation programs for adolescents. *Making Connections*, (Fall): 1-16.

Weiss, H., & Halpern, R. 1991. *Community-based family support and education programs: Something old or something new?* New York, NY: National Center for Children in Poverty, Columbia University.

Weiss, J. A. . 1981. Substance vs. Symbol in administrative reform: The case of human services coordination. *Policy Analysis*, 7: 21-45.

Weissbourd, R. 1991. Making the system work for poor children. *Paper for the Executive Session on Making the System Work for Poor Children.* Cambridge, MA: Harvard University.

Weisz, J.R., Weiss, B., Alicke, M.D., & Klotz, M.L. 1987. Effectiveness of psychotherapy with children and adolescents: A meta-analysis for clinicians. *Journal of Consultative Psychology*, 55: 542-549.

Wells, K., & Biegel, D. 1991. *Family preservation services: Research and evaluation.* Newbury Park, CA: Sage Publications.

Werner, M.J. 1991. Adolescent substance abuse. *Maternal and Child Health Technical Information Bulletin*, 1-16.

Westbrook, L.E., & Stein, R.E.K. 1994. Epidemiology of chronic health conditions in adolescents. In Robert T. Brown and Susan M. Coupey (Eds.), *Adolescent medicine: Chronic and disabling disorders*, 5 (2): 197-210. Philadelphia, PA: Hanley & Belfus, Inc.

White House Conference on Families, The. 1980a. *Listening to America's families: Action for the 80's: The report.* Washington, DC: United States Government Printing Office.

White House Conference on Families, The. 1980b. *Listening to America's families: Action for the 80's: A summary of the report to the President, Congress, and families of the nation.* Washington, DC: United States Government Printing Office.

Whittaker, J.K., Kinney, J., Tracy, E.M., & Booth, C. 1990. *Reaching high-risk families: Intensive family preservation in human services.* New York, NY: Aldine de Gruyter.

Widom, C.S. 1992. The cycle of violence. *National Institute of Justice: Research In Brief*, (October): 1-6.

Willging, J.P., Bower, C.M., & Cotton, R.T. 1992. Physical abuse of children: A retrospective and an otolaryngology perspective. *Arch Otolaryngol Head Neck Surgery*, 118: 247-253.

Williams, B.C., & Kotch, J.B. 1990. Excess injury mortality among children in the United States: Comparison of recent international statistics. *Pediatrics*, 1067-1073.

Williams, H.J., & Waszak, C. 1990. *School-based clinics: Update 1990.* Washington, DC: The Center for Population Options.

Wilmoth, G.H. 1992. Abortion, public health policy, and informed consent legislation. *Journal of Social Issues*, 48: 1-17.

Wilmoth, G.H, de Alteriis, M., & Bussell, D. 1992. Prevelance of psychological risks following legal abortion in the U.S.: Limits of the evidence. *Journal of Social Issues,* 48: 37-66.

Wilson, J.Q. 1991. Character versus intellect: Habits of the heart. *On Character.* Washington, DC: AEI Press.

Wilson, J.Q. 1993. *The moral sense.* New York, NY: The Free Press.

Wilson, W.J. 1991. Public policy research and *the truly disadvantaged.* In Christopher Jencks and Paul E. Peterson (Eds.), *The urban underclass,* pp. 460-482. Washington, DC: Brookings.

Wilson-Brewer, R. 1995. Peer violence prevention programs in middle and high schools. In Katherine Kaufer Christoffel & Carol W. Runyan (Eds.), *Adolescent medicine: Adolescent injuries: Epidemiology and prevention,* 6 (2): 233-250. Philadelphia, PA: Hanley & Belfus, Inc.

Wise, P.H., & Schorr, L. 1992. The neighborhood: Poverty, affluence, and violence. In Melvin D. Levine, William B. Carey, and Allen C. Crocker (Eds.), *Developmental-behavioral pediatrics,* pp. 160-170. Philadelphia, PA: W.B. Saunders Company.

Wood, D.L., Hayward, R.A., Corey, C.R., Freeman, H.E., & Shaprio, M.F. 1990. Access to medical care for children and adolescents in the United States. *Pediatrics,* 86: 666-672.

Worden, J. K., Flynn, B., Geller, B.M., Chen, M., Shelton, L.G., Secker-Walker, R.H., Solomon, D.S., Solomon, L.J., Couchey, S., & Costanza, M. 1988. Development of a smoking prevention mass media program using diagnostic and formative research. *Preventive Medicine,* 17: 531-558.

Wright, R.A. 1993. Community-oriented primary care: The cornerstone of health care reform. *Journal of the American Medical Association,* 269: 2544-2547.

Wu, L.L., & Martinson, B.C. 1993. Family structure and the risk of a premarital birth. *American Sociological Review,* 58: 210-232.

Wynne, E.A. 1986. Transmitting moral values. *Education Digest,* 51: 26-29.

Yamaguchi, K., & Kandel, D. 1987. Drug use and other determinants of premarital pregnancy and its outcome: A dynamic analysis of competing life events. *Journal of Marriage and the Family,* 49: 257-270.

Yarber, W.L., & Parrillo, A.V. 1992. Adolescents and sexually transmitted diseases. *Journal of School Health,* 62: 331-338.

Zabin, L.S. 1990. Adolescent pregnancy: The clinician's role in intervention. *Journal of General Internal Medicine*, 5: 581-588.

Zabin, L.S., & Clark, S. 1981. Why they delay: A study of teenage family planning clinic patients. *Family Planning Perspectives*, 13: 205-217.

Zaslow, M.J., & Takanishi, R. 1993. Priorities for research on adolescent development. *American Psychologist - Special Issue on Adolescence*, 48: 185-192.

Zigler, E., Taussing, C., & Black, K. 1992. A promising preventative for juvenile delinquency. *American Psychologist*, 47: 997-1006.

Zill, N. 1991. *Recent trends in children's physical and mental health.* Testimony Before the Subcommittee on Children, Family, Drugs, and Alcoholism. Washington, DC: United States Senate Committee on Labor and Human Resources.

Zill, N., & Schoenborn, C.A. 1990. *Developmental learning, and emotional problems: Health of our nation's children, U.S.,* 1988. Hyattsville, MD: National Center for Health Statistics.

INDEX